NATIONAL INSTITUTE SOCIAL SERVICES LIBRARY

Volume 10

OLD AGE HOMES

T0362254

OLD AGE HOMES

ROGER CLOUGH

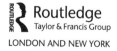
Routledge
Taylor & Francis Group
LONDON AND NEW YORK

First published in 1981 by George Allen & Unwin Ltd

This edition first published in 2022
by Routledge
2 Park Square, Milton Park, Abingdon, Oxon OX14 4RN

and by Routledge
605 Third Avenue, New York, NY 10158

Routledge is an imprint of the Taylor & Francis Group, an informa business

© 1981 Roger Clough

British Library Cataloguing in Publication Data
A catalogue record for this book is available from the British Library

ISBN: 978-1-03-203381-5 (Set)
ISBN: 978-1-00-321681-0 (Set) (ebk)
ISBN: 978-1-03-204314-2 (Volume 10) (hbk)
ISBN: 978-1-03-204318-0 (Volume 10) (pbk)
ISBN: 978-1-00-319142-1 (Volume 10) (ebk)

DOI: 10.4324/9781003191421

Publisher's Note
The publisher has gone to great lengths to ensure the quality of this reprint but points out that some imperfections in the original copies may be apparent.

Disclaimer
The publisher has made every effort to trace copyright holders and would welcome correspondence from those they have been unable to trace.

Old Age Homes

ROGER CLOUGH
Lecturer in Social Work, University of Bristol

London
GEORGE ALLEN & UNWIN
Boston   Sydney

GEORGE ALLEN & UNWIN LTD
40 Museum Street, London WC1A 1LU

© Roger Clough, 1981

British Library Cataloguing in Publication Data

Clough, Roger
    Old age homes. – (National Institute social
    services library; no. 42)
    1. Old age homes – England
    I. Title   II. Series

    ISBN 0-04-362043-4
    ISBN 0-04-362044-2 Pbk

Set in 10 on 11 point Times by Grove Graphics, Tring
and printed in Great Britain
by Richard Clay (The Chaucer Press) Ltd,
Bungay, Suffolk

CONTENTS

Foreword   *page* ix
Acknowledgements   x
Introduction   1
1   Old Age Homes – Myths and Realities   4
2   Styles of Old Age Homes   16
3   Participant Observation in Old Age Homes   30
4   Comparative Background Information   50
5   Going into a Home   63
6   Daily Life for Residents in The Pines   80
7   Mr Jepson and Mrs Williams – Pictures of Two Residents   110
8   Departure   131
9   I Hope We Can Make Them Happy   139
10 Norms and Controls   157
11 Ageing in the Institution   166
12 The Function of Old Age Homes   185
13 The Old: Adults with Rights to Services   202
Appendix 1: Staff Questionnaire   206
Appendix 2: Resident Interview   211
Bibliography   215
Index   219

To my Mother and my Father

FOREWORD

In this disturbing and compassionate book Roger Clough describes the day-to-day life of men and women, residents and staff who live and work at The Pines, an old age home.

He shows the double bind in which residents and staff are enmeshed: a bind created when the prevailing belief that elderly people should keep active is combined with a wish on the part of staff to care for residents and a desire in most old people to be looked after at least to some extent. In demonstrating this situation Roger Clough blames neither staff, residents, nor relatives. All are caught in the confusion in society about the process of ageing and suitable provision for the elderly.

It is appropriate that Roger Clough undertook the participative research for this book when he held a fellowship from the Central Council for Education and Training for Social Work, and that at the time of publication he is a lecturer in a university social work department, because his book demonstrates the value and the possibilities of a social work approach. He shows what an accepting and non-judgemental attitude means in action. He attempts to understand but never to blame and he does not do this from a position of uncertainty or unconcern about what is right for elderly people. That he knows, but he knows too the problems of achieving it.

The book is also a demonstration of the application of the social sciences to the lives of real people and will offer an example to students who find it hard to know the meaning of integrating theory and practice, something which they are exhorted to achieve. They will also learn how to combine feeling and ideas in a way which enriches understanding.

Roger Clough's book is important for its content but also for the way it is written. It illustrates the welding of care and thought which typifies good social work, whether it be research writing, teaching, or practice.

PHYLLIDA PARSLOE
Professor of Social Work,
University of Bristol

Acknowledgment

As a residential practitioner I worked in approved schools with young people (today's community homes with education). My interest in residential work with the elderly developed during several years as a lecturer to students, primarily from old people's homes, on a residential social work course at Bristol Polytechnic. At intervals I would be asked what I really knew or understood about old people's home. And I asked myself what were the similarities and differences between residential work with children and the elderly.

The fellowship awarded to me by the Central Council for Education and Training in Social Work gave me a practical opportunity to examine these questions.

I am grateful to the Council for this opportunity and to those in the Department of Social Sciences in Somerset who agreed to my working in one of the county's homes, in particular to Larry Pritchard and John Fellowes.

Colleagues at Bristol Polytechnic provided me with stimulating supervision during the study period. More recently, when working on this book I have received valuable support, comment and detailed criticism of the text from Christopher Beedell, Roger Bullock, Roy Parker, Phyllida Parsloe and Michael Power at Bristol University. Margaret Windsor has typed both my study notes and the numerous drafts of this book. Phrases like 'residential home' have been written so often that now they type themselves!

Above all my thanks go to the staff and residents of The Pines whom I got to know so well for the way they allowed me to share in their lives. For me, often prone to forget people's names, the vividness with which I can recall not only names but faces, features, expressions and incidents is a testimony to all that my stay at The Pines meant to me.

INTRODUCTION

Two residents of an old people's home, The Pines, describe a typical day.

MISS BRINTON: After breakfast we sit in the lounge and read, have coffee. It's a long period between dinner and tea. When I think of how I used to gallop around! I look forward to visitors, get to know other people's visitors. Bingo seems useless. Here I come up to bed at eight. At home about nine with a milky drink in bed. It takes a long time to get undressed and change the bag [a colostomy bag], one hour or more. I like to do things for myself. I was used to having help with bathing. Here it's more convenient and I'm not embarrassed. At home I had my bath at a regular time from an attendant. Here I have one on the first day and one the last Saturday [she was in for a holiday]. I'm glad to have a bath when it's convenient for the staff but I liked the choice. I'm not rushed – make sure I have long enough – I know I can't do it by myself.

MR MURPHY: It's difficult to get dressed – annoying not being able to tie laces, I don't like having to ask. I usually get up, shave and wash, an 'up and downer'. Get up about five past seven (used to be earlier at home), use a wet razor. I can't see well but it's OK, move off at ten past and down to breakfast at twenty-five past eight. I enjoy the meals, they're good and well cooked – but they give you too much. They can't cook it how you would like it. Usually go up to the sitting room and read the paper. Sleep for half an hour, read the paper, then coffee at eleven. I might move around; go up and down the passage and walk round the place, in the summer I'd go round the garden.

Sit down and talk in my sitting room, never been in other sitting rooms. I know most of them, stop as I go past to talk. The difference isn't the home, the difference is me, can't see well, sight is my biggest loss, gradual loss – had three operations. Came like a yellow blur in the middle of the eye – they operated – and it was worse.

After lunch, sleep, walk, talk, TV and tea. Then
TV again, I stay up until about ten, sometimes nearly
eleven. I get a bit bored in the morning before eleven.
Read the paper and then now't to do. I could go for a
walk but I would be in the way of the cleaners.
Twice a year I go to the British Legion stunt [a
party] – I've got two tickets now but I can't get in
touch with my daughter, I trust her, she's my eyes.
They could phone for me. Don't suppose it would be
difficult to get anyone to write – I'm not much of a one
for asking favours of anyone. When you've lived so
long you're used to doing everything for yourself –
think twice about asking. Sometimes go to bingo. I like
the slide shows and concerts they have.

This book is based on a detailed study of this particular old age home.
It illustrates events and records the feelings, such as those above, of
residents, staff, relatives and other professional groups – doctors,
nurses, health visitors and social workers. Based on this evidence some
explanations are suggested for various patterns of events and some
conclusions are drawn about practice in old age homes.

Old age alters people's pictures of themselves and of life. Two comments from the extracts above illustrate this: 'When I think of how I
used to gallop around', and 'The difference isn't the home, the difference is me'. Each individual is faced with a different set of difficulties
and dilemmas, so there is no single answer to the question 'What is the
secret of a happy or successful old age?'. Nor can a residential home
hope to put right crippling physical or emotional handicaps. What it
should be able to do is to provide a place where an individual's needs
are met in a way that allows her the maximum control of her life.

The first four chapters place such accounts as this in the context of
a wider discussion about residential homes and ageing, together with a
brief discussion of the methods used in this study. From there the bulk
of the book, Chapters 5 to 9, provide the flesh – detailed consideration
of admission and departure, of significant events for staff and residents,
together with a longer study of two residents. The last four chapters
begin the task of considering the relevance of this material to more
general issues – processes of control, ageing in institutions and the objectives of residential establishments.

There are parts of the material that show sadness, harshness and
insensitivity. They are included here not to attack old age homes but
from beliefs that such homes are needed, that they can be good places
to live in and that a clearer understanding of processes that take place
within them is essential.

Finally there are some stylistic points. First, the names of the home and the residents have been altered, though the identity of the residents is maintained. Secondly, since the majority of those in old age homes (staff and residents) are women, I have used feminine pronouns (she, her) rather than the clumsy he/she. It is more difficult to find an adequate title for the place where residents live. 'Old people's home' is the most widely used, though some people refer to 'homes for the elderly' in a belief that the phrase sounds better. 'Home' tells us nothing about the size of the establishment and carries expectations of 'homeliness' which are unrealistic. 'Institution' has overtones of regimentation but may be used in a technical sense to describe an organisation and the building which houses it. Both words – home and institution – will be used in this study to avoid excessive repetition, together with words like centre and establishment. The problem of terminology is more fully discussed elsewhere (Clough 1979a and b).

Chapter 1

OLD AGE HOMES – MYTHS AND REALITIES

Living in an old age home evokes pictures of apathy, dependence and sadness. This is not the image most of us have about our own life in old age. Attitudes seem crystallised in that of Sir Keith Joseph (1972), addressing a one-day conference on residential work, when he looked down from the platform at a group of staff from old age institutions: 'Your old people would rather not be in residential homes, wouldn't they?' he said. Such assumptions, based on the negative aspects of residential homes in general and of old age establishments in particular, have led to policy statements about the desirability of enabling the elderly to stay in their own homes. In this chapter these assumptions are examined and questioned.

ATTITUDES TO AGEING

The starting point is a consideration of attitudes to ageing. Many of the fears that surround old age establishments are in reality fears about old age itself. Old age homes confront us with conspicuous evidence of problems that *may* come with ageing – problems such as confusion, senility, severe and multiple handicap, and the resultant dependence on others. Ten individuals may live in their separate homes sitting for hours doing nothing. If those ten people are grouped together and all seen sitting for hours doing nothing, the image is more than ten times as powerful. No wonder a district nurse responded to a questionnaire by writing:

> The whole aspect of living in an old people's home fills me with horror. The patients appear to me like lodgers in a silent hotel, a place with no pulse, fed, slept and sheltered. Armchairs in rooms, round the edge of the wall, just sitting. The sad thing about the whole thing is that patients sit there from choice . . . I feel they look so pathetic just sitting in silence in armchairs.

Old age is bearable in prospect as long as we can maintain a picture of contentment and continued interest in the world around, and as long as physical or mental impairment does not hit too hard. It is difficult to maintain a picture of successful ageing when some or all of these factors do not apply. The old age home presents society with the apathy or handicap of residents *en masse*. It is easy to forget that old age anywhere may be as unpleasant. Similarly by focusing on the poverty of the life of some residents it is easy to put aside our anxieties about our own old age.

Anxiety about old age has two important aspects: physical deterioration which may affect body or mind; and purposelessness resulting from loss of role, death of friends or relatives, poverty and isolation. Both aspects, physical deterioration or purposelessness, may occur inside or outside a residential home.

To ignore this is to fall into the trap of distorting the reality of old age. An American writer, Gubrium (1973), calls this process 'The myth of the golden years'. A part of this myth concerns the social context of old age. One view of this social context 'is that of the alleged well-being of old people who continue to maintain their own neighbourhood household . . . The first of these images . . . conceives of a self-sufficient couple in an older neighbourhood of homes, who maintain a mutually satisfactory round of daily life. Both are portrayed as actively involved in a variety of crafts and hobby-like activities. Both maintain active local connections in neighbourhoods that are "just as I remember them".'

Gubrium continues, 'Not only are social contexts considered felicitous but so are the relationships between old people as well as their activity. Four images of interaction and activity should be noted: (1) the idea of growing old together; (2) the indulgent intergenerational portrayal of the aged; (3) the ideal active "busyness" of the elderly; and (4) the simple advice of planning for retirement.'

Gubrium explodes the myth – many old people are not in their own neighbourhoods or surrounded by a network of relationships. They may have been rehoused, living in lodgings or flats. The myth ignores the movement of neighbours and the crime rate that leaves the old too frightened to leave their homes. Finally, many old are single, do not get on well with their children and do not have the resources of money or health to remain 'busy' in old age.

It will be apparent later that most professional workers, when considering their own old age in response to questionnaires, thought in terms of the freedom old age would bring and greater opportunities to pursue interests. This is a very important side of old age, rightly stressed by organisations for the aged. But the other side of the coin is weariness and bitterness.

A part of Gubrium's attack is directed against what has been termed the *activity theory* of ageing. This theory, associated particularly with

Havighurst (see Havighurst and Albrecht, 1953), proposes that old people age successfully if society accepts the value of the old and ascribes them publicly valued roles. In particular old people should substitute new activities in old age for those which they give up on retirement. An offshoot of this idea is the claim that people need to plan for old age, which has led to the development of pre-retirement classes to encourage such planning.

Gubrium criticises activity theory on the grounds that activity is seen mostly in terms of work-like situations that are active and visible, and stereotypically middle class. The quality of social relationships is ignored. In addition the high degree of physical dependence and the limited roles available to old people are not examined. It became apparent that some people with high morale had low activity.

An alternative understanding of needs in old age was introduced by Cumming and Henry (1961). They suggested, in what has been termed the *disengagement theory*, that society withdraws from the older person. The individual co-operates in a process of disengagement between himself and society. This is a mutual process. Happiness in old age depends on the individual and society accepting this role for the elderly. While disengagement theory takes into account the needs of society for younger, more active people to replace the older, it may ignore the needs of the elderly. In particular it assumes that this process must take place for all societies and all individuals within that society.

A more recent theme in research work into ageing has been to consider the basis on which one can assess life satisfaction in old age. Havighurst (1968) shows how emphasis has shifted away from the either/or debate surrounding the conflict between the activity and disengagement theories. Citing the Kansas City Study of Adult Life he states (p. 304):

> The results of this study indicated that neither the activity nor the disengagement theory was adequate to account for the observed facts. While there was a decrease of engagement in the common social roles related to increasing age, some of the people who remained active and engaged showed a high degree of satisfaction. On the whole those who were most active at the older ages were happier, but there were many exceptions to this rule.

This study carried on the work of others in looking for a personality dimension as a factor that influenced successful ageing. An analysis was produced which was based on three dimensions – personality, role activity and life satisfaction. Havighurst concludes (p. 308):

> Of the three dimensions on which we have data – activity, satisfaction and personality – personality seems to be the pivotal dimension

in describing patterns of ageing and in predicting relationships between level of activity and life satisfaction.

In contrast Gubrium, in his socio-environmental approach, emphasises the interplay of two factors – activity resources and activity norms. Activity resources are those resources which enable a person to do the things she wishes. They include money, housing, local facilities, social support and health. Activity norms are the norms that an individual has come to accept and share in common with others about what she should be doing.

This theory stresses the importance to old people of expectations about activity. The old will be satisfied when they are able to do what they and others regard as appropriate. Mr Murphy (p. 1 above) found his health worse – he was nearly blind and could move only with difficulty. Yet he did not like having to ask other people to tie his shoe laces. So his resources did not match his norms. Gubrium argues that someone may be said to be coping or have high morale when her resources match the norms set by herself and others. The theory is particularly helpful in explaining why many residents at The Pines found it hard to adjust to their worsening physical state.

Thus attitudes to old age institutions are influenced by fears about old age itself. In addition there is no agreement about what constitutes or results in successful old age. The old may not have the resources to match expectations and, while it is possible to envisage providing the old with more money or better facilities, it is unlikely that much can be done about deterioration in health. Consequently it is necessary to adjust norms as well as to look for better resources.

ATTITUDES TO RESIDENTIAL LIVING

Old age homes have similarities to organisations like homes for the physically handicapped or long-stay hospitals in which residents are expected to be permanent. Yet all such organisations, along with most other residential establishments, are regarded as second best to living in one's own home. There are only a few exceptions. In situations where there is a high degree of voluntary entry to establishments (i.e. there are several other living styles available and the residential home is the preferred choice) or where great importance is attached to the purpose for entry (e.g. boarding school) residential living is seen more favourably. Religious establishments, hotels, communes and boarding schools come into this category. Social service type institutions – for children, the mentally or physically ill, the mentally or physically handicapped, the old – fall into the second-best category. The negative aspects of such establishments have been well documented and have become part of the conventional wisdom. Residential institutions have been criticised for almost as long as they have been in existence. Criticism has been intense since the 1950s. Bowlby (1951) cited the dangers for children in institutions from maternal deprivation. Barton (1959) stated that living in institutions could produce a set of problems (which he called institutional neurosis) more difficult to eradicate than the original reason for admission. Goffman, in a series of major essays brought together in *Asylums* (1961), discussed the totality and pervasiveness of institutional regimes. The more total the regime, the more an institution devised rituals to ensure that physical constraints (such as walls and locked doors) were matched by social pressures to conformity and he illustrated this theme by examining the 'stripping' of the person that took place at admission.

With this as background has followed a succession of studies of types of institution – for example, Townsend (1962) on old people's homes, Morris and Morris (1963) on Pentonville, Morris (1969) on subnormality hospitals, Meacher (1972) about homes for the elderly confused. These have added their weight to the criticism of residential institutions.

ATTITUDES TO OLD AGE HOMES

Today's elderly have vivid memories of the workhouse, the predecessor of local authority old people's homes. The workhouse has become a symbol of harsh, unimaginative and regimented living. Whether such a picture is true or not, the tradition lives on. The old consider entering a residential home to be a sign of failure and, on admission, expect to be compliant.

Townsend's study was a significant landmark in the development of attitudes to old age homes. After the Second World War there were hopes that new and smaller residential homes would lead to more satisfactory living conditions for the elderly. Townsend showed the inadequacy of building programmes but also the inadequacy of life-style within many purpose-built establishments. The view of the old age home as second best was reinforced.

The Williams Committee (1967), set up to examine the training needs of staff in residential homes and acknowledge the importance and the skill of the work, expressed similar sentiments:

> One basic fact has to be kept in mind, that even the best residential home is likely to be ranked as second best in the mind of those who come into it. It cannot replace the independence a person enjoys in his own home or give what an affectionate family can provide. Everything is different from what he has been accustomed to for so long. The rooms may be warm and bright and prettily decorated, the chairs comfortable, the food good and plentiful. But they are

different and take getting used to. And one's new companions are not those whom one has known all one's life, who understand the names that crop up in the conversation or recognise the references to past experiences. It is a sad thing not only to suffer the infirmities of old age but to find oneself among strangers at a time of life when it is difficult to make new friends.

Not surprisingly there have been demands to put resources into 'community' and 'preventive' work, though I have argued elsewhere that this contrast between 'residential home' and 'community' is inaccurate and unhelpful, for residential establishments are very much part of the community (see Clough, 1978a).
Townsend (1962) suggests

a number of far-reaching proposals . . . to reduce progressively the number of communal homes (in the first instance by closing the former workhouses) and to replace them in part by sheltered housing and in part by a slight extension of the hospital system . . . to enlarge greatly the domiciliary services, mainly by creating a local authority family help service, and to develop general practitioner group practices.

Meacher (1969) argues for a similar change of policy:

The Government should declare an unequivocal commitment to reverse the emphasis of social policy in old age from care in institutions to care in the wider community. This should be based not only on considerations of cost-effectiveness or on the well documented pathologies of institutional life, but on the urgent need to give priority to developing preventive services and to keeping the individual within the therapeutic framework of the family circle and the surrounding network of friends and neighbours, with its interchange of services between generations.

So the stereotype became established that people, whether young or old, mentally ill or subnormal, were better off in their own homes. Residential institutions have been regarded as evils, whether necessary or unnecessary evils.

'Of course there are some exceptions; but in the main the conditions of our residential institutions are appalling.' This statement from a *Guardian* editorial (27 January 1978) typifies this attitude, as does a report by Conrad Jamieson for Cheshire Social Services in 1973:

On the surface an old age home might seem to be only a geriatric ward in disguise. The picture it presents is all too often one of dependency, discouragement, confusion and the regressive and senile behaviour of second childhood. Yet below the surface is an unrealised potential for the institutionalised old to live normal, healthy and self-sufficient lives. Why isn't this potential being better realised even in well run and modern homes . . . ?

The symptoms of senility which proliferate in old age homes cannot be put down as due solely to the ageing process, but must be attributed largely to the institution of the old age home itself in creating what we call 'situational senility' which is induced by a particular set of environmental factors. The harsh truth would seem to be that residents of old age homes do not grow senile in spite of institutionalisation but because of it. Two factors in particular would seem to explain situational senility:

(a) the forcibleness of the uprooting the old person undergoes in entering a home

(b) the role expectations within the home itself which covertly or overtly encourage dependent and regressive behaviour.

In the *Guardian* was the comment on this report: 'even the most modern home schemes offer little hope of mitigating the effects of institutionalisation to any appreciable degree. The resident often enters a home in a demoralised state, feeling rejected by family or friends with whom it will be difficult to maintain relationships'.

The potential dangers are magnified by an awareness of the high degree of dependence of residents and the possibility of maladministration and cruelty by those running the home. Numerous examples could be given of inefficiency and cruelty in a range of residential establishments. In old age homes one illustration of violence was the conviction of a superintendent for assaults on residents. Witnesses stated:

The residents sat in the same chairs, they were not allowed to do anything for themselves. They were like robots.

[His] attitude to patients made them subdued and crestfallen.

The superintendent pinned a resident in his chair against the table and yanked back his head and pushed food into his mouth, at the same time shouting at him. This was an unpardonable and unlawful use of force [the prosecution claimed].

Mr (M) would not always move his legs. [His] reaction was to kick him on the legs to make him walk. One mealtime he fell on the floor. As he lay there on the floor [he] kicked him on the top of his legs. (Extracts from *Oxford Mail*, 1973)

Any suggestion that residential care could be beneficial has, by comparison, been slight. Discussion of such benefits as have been mentioned has been primarily in relation to treatment-oriented units, especially with young people. But Harris (1968) states that a large majority of the residents of old age homes enjoy living in the home. Simpson (1971) examines the implications of the different regimes of three old age homes and concludes that one style of living is preferable because it produces mobile, physically active and social residents. Most recently Brearley (1977), though accepting that the best residential home will be second best in the mind of the individual, stresses that 'work with the elderly can be interesting, worthwhile and successful'.

DOMICILIARY OR RESIDENTIAL CARE

Righton (1977) makes a similar point.

Catalogues of the disadvantages of residential care are all too common: often compiled by academic psychologists and sociologists whose experience of communal living is remarkable chiefly for its brevity, they are usually referred to collectively in articles and lecture halls as the 'literature of dysfunction'. Lists of advantages, by contrast, are as rare as air on the top of Mount Everest, and about as invigorating.

There is no doubt of the potential dangers in residential care but there are potential dangers in families and in living! There is too often a facile assumption that domiciliary services are by nature superior. In the same way anything that can claim to be 'preventive' may enhance its legitimation. If the dangers and also the cost inherent in residential care are put in the background, an important question can emerge. Are cruelty and regimentation inevitable factors of residential living or are they examples of bad practice? Put the other way this becomes – is there anything intrinsic about residential homes to suggest that living in a well-run residential home is not as adequate as living in a well-run home in the wider community?

There are fallacies in the belief that for *all* people, at *all* times, living in the wider community is preferable. This stereotype is supported by a number of assumptions. The first of these places an idealised model of domiciliary care alongside a picture of inadequate residential care.

The strengths of domiciliary care – the maintenance of an established pattern of life, the 'normality' of living – are seen in ideal terms. This means that the inherent possibilities domiciliary services could provide for some are assumed to be available, functional and appropriate to all. This is contrasted with 'the well-known pathologies of residential life' (Meacher, 1969), in other words the problems inherent in residential living – loss of freedom to make decisions, loss of independence, loss of one's own home, isolation. In fact the existing model is contrasted with the ideal and the conclusion that the ideal is best is not surprising.

It would be as easy to do the reverse procedure. One could discuss residential homes in ideal terms – as being therapeutic communities that enable the elderly to lead fuller lives – and contrast this with the squalor, the deprivation, the apathy, the lack of relationships and the failure of domiciliary services outside them. Such a study could show that meals on wheels are too rushed, too infrequent and often thrown away; that social workers, health visitors and doctors have been 'unable to spot and ensure treatment of the miseries of old age' (Goldberg, 1970); that visits by volunteers are irregular and patronising; that in spite of the mobilisation of considerable resources many old people remain lonely, friendless and isolated. Either method of idealising one type of provision and comparing this with an existing service is mistaken.

Another assumption is that 'home is always best'. The belief in the superiority of home life seems based on the fact that it is the norm. But this does not mean that this ought to be the accepted pattern for everybody. Indeed, we may well be moving into an age when the isolation of the family is rejected more often in favour of communal living. Living on one's own is not necessarily better than living with other people.

A very real danger of present research is that it accepts the present norms and attempts to provide substitutes for them. Thus we attempt to substitute 'residential care' for 'home life' and we assess the adequacy of residential care by the degree to which it approaches the norm of home life. The basic assumptions themselves need questioning – in this case that home is always best – and in particular one has to examine whether an individual has ever lived according to the norm.

Of course, home is the best for some people. Just because that statement is so obviously true one must be on one's guard against presuming it is true for everybody. Many old people may never find real warmth, real nurture and care and real friendship while living in their own homes. This may be so whatever quantity, quality and type of domiciliary services are offered, for it is doubtful if such services can ever supply such needs. Some old people may be loved and cherished in the setting of a residential home in a way that is not possible in any other type of care. The very 'residentialness', to use a clumsy word, which involves physical caring and the supplying of emotional needs is obviously applicable only to the residential home.

Of course, physical needs can be met in such a way that emotional needs are not fulfilled. Food can be served so sloppily that it is clear that the cook has no interest in the person for whom the food is provided; but equally presentation of food can demonstrate the warmth of the caring relationship. So living in a residential unit may supply the needs of some old people.

There are other strengths to residential work which could be singled out – twenty-four-hour observation and care, an ability to deal with the rapid change in feeling on top of the world or under the weather that old people face, a greater likelihood of lending support in the many aspects of loss that have to be faced, a chance for the resident to do more because some of the problems of living are removed, the probability that the miseries of old age will be better cared for.

It is important in this context to realise that many of the old people at present in residential care are those who have been unable to sustain a normal pattern of relationships at home. So it is unreasonable to judge the residential unit solely by the degree to which normal relationships appear to exist.

Another aspect of this discussion is cost-effectiveness. Residents in old age institutions are becoming older and more dependent at admission. Their needs are considerable and to meet such needs adequately via domiciliary services would necessitate a vast growth in such services. Domiciliary provision for the highly dependent is only cheaper while it is less adequate – while it fails to provide twenty-four-hour cover, laundry services, regular meals, help with bathing, toileting, housework, cooking. The list could be immense (Hobman, 1977).

THE INTERTWINING OF TWO MYTHS

The two myths –the myth of the golden years and the myth of the evil institution – when intertwined appear to present an irrefutable argument that the old are best kept out of unpleasant residential homes to live an active and fulfilled life from their own home base. Limits and provisos must be placed on such a statement.

The prevailing attitude, that stresses the limitations or even harmful effects of residential care, is sustained by many who are not in a situation where they have to make a choice about living arrangements in old age. It may well be that, with family around and strong neighbourhood ties, a residential home seems abhorrent; is it so abhorrent when one is old and lonely with many friends already dead? Indeed, how many people making the sort of statements that are made about inadequate residential care are faced with the emotional deprivation of cooking or cleaning only for oneself after having done this for a family?

Another aspect of the 'golden years myth' is the esteem given to independence. It seems widely accepted that one of the virtues of domiciliary care is that it encourages old people to do things for themselves and the principle is becoming accepted for residential care as well. Of course, independence and self-help are important goals. But they should not be over-riding goals. The morality of encouraging some old people to go on struggling through most of their waking day to do little other than maintain themselves and the fabric of their environment should be questioned. Outsiders, even families, may believe it is right to persuade the old to carry on in their own homes. Mrs Richardson (p. 65 below) describes how the household tasks had got too much and she was relieved to be cared for, even though she was now farther from her family.

Peter Townsend (1962) lists nine fundamental principles which might be embodied in 'a realistic and enlightened general policy for the aged'. His fourth principle is that an individual should be helped 'to live as independently as possible in a home of his own'. His commitment to the value of domiciliary care means that the *potential* of the residential home is ignored. Two further sentences highlight this: 'On the available evidence we are obliged to conclude reluctantly that the residential home, at least as it has taken shape in the post-war years, is misconceived and inappropriate. It does not fit rationally into a coherent system of services for the elderly and handicapped.' While it is important to examine the significance of Townsend's survey of what life was like for residents of old people's homes, it is not necessary to adopt the conclusion that resources should be shifted to domiciliary services.

The problem for old age homes is compounded because of uncertainty about their purpose. Should they be the 'hotels for pensioners' of Aneurin Bevan's dreams or are they better seen as special housing provision? In addition there is far less clarity about normal patterns of caring for the old than about child-rearing. Adults have lived through childhood; adults are usually available to rear children and the norms of such rearing would command wide acceptance. By contrast those planning provision for the old have not been old themselves; families may not be available to provide care, and the old, with adult responsibility for choice of life-style that is not given to children, will present a greater scatter of views (Clough, 1978b).

Townsend uses his analysis of the shortcomings of residential institutions to propose major changes in provision. By contrast Goldberg (1970), while illustrating the failures of social workers, spells out the implications of her research for the task of the field worker. It is similarly possible to consider the shortcomings of residential work *and* the implications for the task to be performed. Until this is done the quality of work with the elderly will be the poorer.

Homes for the elderly are in existence; demand for them is increasing faster than provision. These residential homes will remain in existence for the forseeable future. Whether or not they are ideal living situations, they are necessary ones. Constant denial of the value of their task will lead to a further lowering of the morale of staff. As a first step to improving morale and consequently the life-style and happiness of those within the homes it is essential that a clearer understanding be developed of the processes in an old age home.

Margaret Tilley (1971) suggests that happiness is the main objective of a residential home and that the home which promotes this is indeed a therapeutic community. She continues: 'It is worth noting that in work with the aged one can be an uninhibited hedonist, for, unlike children, their characters are made or marred and one does not have to take into account character formation.'

Earlier in her paper she writes: 'Perhaps more than anything, at this present stage of development in residential provision for the elderly, we need some imaginative and exploratory thinking so that we can ask the right questions about old people's needs and wishes as a necessary preliminary to discovering how these can best be met.'

This study is an attempt to ask the right questions about old people's needs. It shows daily happenings within one home and offers explanations for some of these events. Where there is dissatisfaction with the life-style that is portrayed, whether dissatisfaction of reader or author, such feeling may be a spur to finding more appropriate ways of meeting the needs of the elderly within a residential home.

Chapter 2

STYLES OF OLD AGE HOMES

There are so many assumptions about the elderly that it is essential to be able to place them in a context. The typology of old age homes that is introduced (p. 22 below) allows events to be examined in relation to specified variables. Such a framework is valuable but must not lead to oversimplification. One of the major goals of social research should be to avoid simplistic explanations (see pp. 18–19 below). In the first part of this chapter I give the rationale for the framework developed later.

ATTITUDES TO AGEING: 'IT'S FOR THEIR GOOD'

One of the aspects of residential homes that I find disturbing is the ease with which it is possible for staff, especially senior staff, to translate their attitudes into action. One matron explained to me that her residents were given margarine rather than butter because it was better for their health; another served an afternoon cup of tea only to those able to walk to the dining room because activity was good for them. It is by this most seductive phrase that the lives of many old people are ruled. The old, in and out of residential homes, are advised to drink more or to drink less, to keep active, to get out, to get up and to eat up because *it is good for them*. So the whims and fancies of staff are readily translated into action. I was anxious to find out what were the beliefs of the staff and residents about the appropriate styles of living. How far could such attitudes be linked to particular assumptions about the ageing process?

The uncertainties as to what constitutes successful ageing have already been mentioned. They are of particular importance here. In caring for children, adults draw on their own experience of being a child; in caring for the old there is no first-hand experience. No wonder some old people insisted staff did not know 'what it is like to be old'. Comments from residents such as 'They'll understand when they are old that old people must not be rushed' were frequent.

In addition there is less written about the needs of the old than those of children. In residential child care part of the task is to provide the resources for healthy development in the light of knowledge available about children's needs. This is an aspect of what Beedell (1970) calls 'parenting'. He states that parenting involves 'holding', 'nurturing' and 'provision for the development and maintenance of personal integrity'. There is no word to describe the task of 'parenting your elders' but, even were such a word available, there is little analysis of what the components of that task should be. For example, Beedell states about nurturing: 'All societies have arrangements for encouraging, and sometimes insisting on the development of skills; social, physical and intellectual.' Such a global statement could not be made about nurturing the elderly.

It is, of course, arguable that residential care of the elderly should take as its prime task the holding aspect of provision. 'All societies have customs and rituals designed to ensure the dependent child's survival and to protect him from danger, discomfort and distress. In doing so they give the child mainly good experiences of care, comfort and control' (Beedell, 1970). Yet, while 'holding' is an essential aspect of the task of caring for the old, it should not become the only one. The elderly have nurturing and development needs also. The body of knowledge of what constitutes such needs is minimal. Consequently individual assumptions are likely to play a larger part in meeting such needs.

A BROAD EXPLANATION OF EVENTS

It is at this stage that it is necessary to repeat the statement that old age institutions are an integral part of the community. Many studies have examined residential institutions as separate entities. Morris (1969), by contrast, makes the point: 'However much it may appear so from the inside, subnormality hospitals are not islands unto themselves, but are a part of a wider community.' Attitudes of staff and residents are not formed in isolation. Consequently it was decided for this study to include an assessment of the attitudes of people outside the institution – in this case field social workers, doctors, health visitors, district nurses and relatives of residents.

So one part of the picture presented here is drawn around attitudes to ageing. Another part shows attitudes to residential living. If residential homes are regarded as second best and less than adequate, in particular if entry to a residential home is regarded as failure, then it would not be surprising to discover that residents found the life dissatisfying. This fact has been demonstrated in other situations. Miller and Gwynne (1972) argue in relation to homes for the disabled that residents may be 'socially dead' before admission. The inability to fulfil roles such as breadwinner and husband is itself a sign of failure. Entry to a residential home only confirms an existing situation. Tobin and Lieberman (1976) show how acknowledgement that one is going to enter into a residential home is a key factor in apathy within a residential home. In other words entry to a residential institution confirms the perception of oneself as an individual without valid social roles. Passivity and dependence comes from the process that *precedes* admission as well as that which takes place after entry to a home. An example from my own study illustrates this (Clough, 1978c):

Mrs Smith had lived in a sheltered housing scheme prior to admission to an old people's home. She described to me her life, entertaining the family, and her involvement in a wide range of activities. She was a lively member of a local church, baked more cakes for the coffee morning than anyone else and had a positive picture of her past. Within the residential home her life had changed – physically, since bouts of arthritis left her crippled and in severe pain on occasion; spiritually, since she could no longer believe in a God who had allowed so much to happen to her; socially, for she had cut off links with her church and past friends. She did retain close links with her family and, though she described herself as bitter, kept going at some things such as knitting . . .

The temptation is to consider that these situations arise from the ill effects of institutional living. The dreaded institutionalisation has struck again! Such an explanation is far too simple. It presumes that the ill effects arise from institutional life, whereas there may be other significant factors.

Mrs Smith's life prior to admission to a residential home was very full. Her life after admission was not. It is in such situations that institutionalisation is so seductive an explanation. However, her change in attitude and life-style is much better explained by the anticipation of living in a home. She was clear that living in a residential home was a visible indication of one's reduced purpose in society. Her response to this was to initiate the severing of past ties. It was her assumptions about the status of residents in old age homes that led to her bitterness. *The actual life-style within the home was not the reason for her change in attitude.*

A second example illustrates the way that the feeling of rejection by one's family plays a significant part in life within the institution (Clough, 1978c).

By contrast, Mrs Draxton appeared to have given up. Her moaning and complaints were constant – she was bored but felt there was nothing else to do. She sat and sat; residents and staff tried to arouse her interest but gave up, discouraged. Again, this was a contrast to her former life, struggling to educate her daughter as a doctor, taking pride in her ability at crafts. Her daughter, with whom she had been living, was going to move away; the daughter thought her mother would be better off in a residential home. Mrs Draxton was still bemused when I met her, months after admission, as to why she needed to be in a home and how she had got there. She was facing loss and a major break in the continuity of her life.

THE FUNCTIONS OF RESIDENTIAL ESTABLISHMENTS

One of the ways in which I tried to draw some of these threads together was to consider different approaches to running old age homes.

Goffman (1961), in his study of total institutions, listed five categories:

(1) institutions established to care for persons felt to be incapable and harmless; these are the homes for the blind, the aged, the orphaned and the indigent;
(2) institutions for those who are incapable but comprise an unintended threat to society;
(3) institutions for the protection of society from intended danger;
(4) institutions for the transmission of work-like skills;
(5) institutions for those wishing to retreat from society.

Moss (1975) has a different set of functions:

healing;
compensation for deprivation or disablement;
acquisition of certain common social skills/habits;
the facilitation of certain work or the acquisition of special roles or skills;
the acquisition of caste/class/party values and habits;
deterrence or punishment;
protection of the community from 'harmful' influences;
protection of inmates from corruption, exploitation;
elimination or neutralisation of inmates.

Meacher (1972) discusses more specifically the functions of separatism in social policy. He reviews a wide range of institutions and considers to whom the benefits of such separatism accrue. Such segregation, he argues, needs to be understood in terms of the interests of the beneficiaries of dissociation. For example, the remainder of society benefits from prisons, rich and powerful families from public schools. He continues:

Since then segregation is by nature manipulative, however indirectly, it follows that, except where it is exercised voluntarily and the beneficiaries of dissociation are identical to those to whom it is applied, its consequences are likely to be at best limiting and at worst punitive.

Meacher uses this as a basis for examining special residential homes for the confused elderly. There are similar important questions about the functions of other old age institutions. Who profits from such establishments, what types of selection and restriction exist, in what ways does segregation take place?

Old age institutions do not fit readily into any of Moss's categories though they may be thought of as providing compensation for deprivation, or healing. They are mentioned specifically in the first of Goffman's groupings: 'institutions caring for persons felt to be incapable and harmless'. On the sort of analysis used by Meacher it is possible to suggest that they benefit relatives and younger able-bodied people, that restrictions are in terms of indefinite residential living because no other alternative is possible.

The functions of the old age home are significant, for greater clarity is needed about the tasks it carries out. In addition it is apparent that it is easier to assess whether some functions are satisfactorily fulfilled than others. There is a variety of ways of assessing whether schools have transmitted instrumental skills successfully, of which the most obvious is to assess examination results.. Similarly it is possible to see whether prisons can contain prisoners without escapes, whether isolation hospitals prevent the spread of disease; even when considering establishments such as community homes and special schools, when goals are less certain, it is possible to look at factors such as integration with family and community, academic achievements, social achievements, ability to 'survive' without recourse to welfare establishments.

Indeed, much recent writing has stressed measurement, whether of behaviour ratings of children in the Measure of Treatment Potential or the linking of staff–child interaction with performance in tests of reading and arithmetic in units for autistic children (Grygier, Bartak and Rutter, 1975). In this way it is possible to discover which regime will lead to an increase in the achievement of the child.

Without the end measurement (in this example the performance tests) it is less easy to use any scales that may be devised. It is the lack of measurable objectives that make long-term caring institutions for adults difficult to assess.

Far more account has to be taken of the extent to which the individual resident is satisfied with his current life-style and the service provided. Though there may be severe financial limitations it may be possible to demonstrate that one regime produces more satisfied residents than another; alternatively it may be possible to show that particular regimes produce particular results and then to allow a moral decision about which regime and result is preferred. Pincus (1968) devised a framework for studying the institutional environment. He developed a questionnaire which was designed to provide information on four dimensions: (1) public–private; (2) structured–unstructured; (3) resource sparse–resource rich; (4) isolated–integrated.

The theme of assessment of residential homes is taken up in two recent publications, Peace, Hall and Hamblin (1979) and Hughes and Wilkin (1980). The first group of authors look for a 'quality of life' rating which draws on the experience of consumers. The second publication, while accepting 'quality of life' as a useful scale, points out the limitations of such an approach, particularly if it relies too heavily on a group of consumers who are likely to be uncritical.

Probably it is better to search for the components of 'quality of life' rather than to attempt a composite score. This will allow comparison between establishments on a range of variables, as would Pincus's questionnaire, but would not presume that there is certainty about how to score any characteristic. For example, it is useful to know that residents in one home spend more time sitting in a lounge than in another. But it must be remembered that any individual may wish to spend more or less time in the lounge. There is no right amount of public living.

MODELS IN RESIDENTIAL INSTITUTIONS

Essentially the move to identify models in residential institutions has developed from a wish to identify characteristics and so to chart different styles of home, with implications about the impact on residents and staff. It is perhaps part of a movement that has looked for variations other than the extent to which an institution is more or less total.

So Miller and Gwynne (1972) hypothesise three models – warehousing, horticultural and organisational – in homes for physically handicapped adults. The first is linked to 'the humanitarian defence' in which 'humanitarian values apply pressure to postpone physical death for as long as possible' though the unhappiness of those whose life is prolonged may be unacknowledged. The horticultural is linked to 'the liberal defence' – 'the abnormality of the inmates is denied: it is claimed that they are 'really normal . . . by treating such a person as normal the abnormality, with its limitations, is denied.' The third model is based on a belief that the task of the organisation is to support the individual in the choice he has made about life-style. 'He may choose dependence, he may choose hyperactivity; he may modify his choice as his physical condition changes.' Whichever he chooses, the task of the organisation is to support that choice.

This approach is a base for that of Meacher (1972), who posits four models based on different philosophies: (1) euthanasia; (2) warehousing; (3) horticulture; (4) social deprivation. Only the fourth needs any elaboration. This is based on his tenet that since part of 'the causation of mental confusion among the aged entails a strong social component', then compensation should be a major factor to encourage full integration and normalisation.

Millham, Bullock and Cherrett (1975a) and Moss (1975) provide two other examples. Millham and colleagues in a study of approved schools suggest different styles of school – nautical school, senior training school, junior training school, family group school, campus school therapeutic community. They proceed to illustrate the differences in type of philosophy, organisation, systems of control and other factors.

Moss (1975) builds, perhaps, on the work of King, Raynes and Tizard (1971) who have suggested that medical and child care outlooks lead to different life-styles for institutions. Moss lists three main models – child care, educational, medical/nursing – while a fourth model, housing, ought to but does not exist in any numbers. He lists a variety of factors such as size and siting of unit, type of staff and children, and compares the differences with these three models.

TYPOLOGY OF OLD AGE INSTITUTIONS

However, work on old people's homes has, by comparison, been minimal and heavily dependent on a survey of institutions for old people by Townsend (1962). Part of the reason for this present study was to consider what may be important variables in different life-styles for old people in institutions.

Table 2.1 *Typology of Old Age Institutions*

CONTROL OF LIFE-STYLE BY RESIDENT	Model of Ageing		
	Activity	*Disengagement*	*Socio-environmental*
Minimal control by resident	(1) Nursing home	(4) Institution	(7) 'Home'
Some control	(2) Therapeutic unit	(5) Hotel	(8) Hostel
Maximum feasible control	(3) Retirement community	(6) Flatlets	(9) Supportive unit

The typology I have used (Table 2.1) is developed from two variables: (1) the extent to which a resident controls her life-style; (2) different models of ageing. Its value is in the extent to which it makes *explicit* some of the assumptions which are often hidden. The names are chosen to indicate a style of life within an institution. Thus the table allows comparison between a 'nursing home' style and a 'hotel' style of institution, but I am not suggesting that all nursing homes or all hotels conform to these styles.

The models in the table illustrate some of the patterns of living that various combinations of these two variables may produce. Such models are devised as ways of describing regimes more precisely and allow for individual choice as to the most appropriate style of living.

The models are discussed in detail below. The following factors were used to compare institutions: (1) type of admission (the degree of control by the resident and others); (2) theories and assumptions about ageing; (3) aims of organisations; (4) staffing implications (staff–resident ratio, authority structures, use of uniforms, job demarcation); (5) building implications (block or units, types of lounges); (6) control systems (regulations, formal and informal expectations); (7) control of life-style by resident (indicators used – money, cleaning, daily programme, bathing, medicines and drugs, meals, furniture and decorating). The same outline is used subsequently for the study of the particular home in this study, The Pines. The details below are hypothetical outlines.

There are limitations to this approach. The precision that such an analysis may suggest cannot be wholly upheld. Institutions may fit broadly into one of these categories but the large numbers of personnel involved (staff, residents, outsiders) will not all have the same assumptions about the ageing process. Indeed, that is one of the major problems for residents who may have different assumptions from those of staff. The 'model of ageing' variable is used to indicate the predominant attitude within the institution, which is likely to be that of the staff. There are further limitations to the use of these theories. In particular a key part of the disengagement theory is that the process of disengagement involves co-operation between the individual and society. So 'disengagement' is used here to indicate a predominant attitude that the process of withdrawal from active roles is the key to successful ageing. The way in which such a view may be imposed on others is a separate, though important, question. This would relate to life inside or outside a residential establishment and is discussed by Lowenthal and Boler (1965), though not in relation to residential institutions.

Brief synopses of all nine styles of old age institutions are given below, while four styles (the nursing home, therapeutic unit, institution and supportive unit) are developed in greater detail.

The first three types are based on an activity theory of ageing. This postulates that successful ageing involves finding replacement activities for those that are given up through retirement or ill-health.

(1) *Nursing home*
This is a staff-dominated establishment with prevailing beliefs that limbs need to be exercised; that people need to be taken out of themselves, that residents, if left alone, will become apathetic.

Many residents will have been transferred from hospital; residents are thought to need residential care because they are not fit enough to manage outside. 'They will keep you going and keep you young' residents will be told.

Stress is placed on the efficiency of the unit and on planning activities rather than the happiness or satisfaction of the residents.

A hierarchical system exists with the head known as 'Matron'; staff are nurse trained and wear uniforms; there is clear job demarcation. The building is large, necessitating much communal activity, and there are few single rooms.

Staff and residents are aware of strict rules. They are enforced by physical constraints, for example, removal of cigarettes, forced feeding, manhandling to bath, control of places of seating and sleeping, threat of transfer.

Residents have minimal control over their life-style. Pension books are held centrally. Residents are given money rarely; it is spent for them. There is great emphasis on cleaning and hygiene, with thorough cleaning of rooms every day; the more active residents are given tasks. Stress is placed on routines, and residents are expected to conform; they must join in with activities arranged for them; activities are valued because they keep people occupied. There is a fixed bath rota with close supervision by staff. All residents have the same doctor; staff call the doctor when they think necessary; staff keep and distribute all drugs. Meals are held at set times; residents must attend, must eat something and have no choice; the feeble or unwilling may be forcibly fed. Rooms are seen as belonging to the organisation; residents have no say in their decor, and few possessions around; staff enter rooms without knocking and will put away items they do not wish to have around; furniture and floor coverings may be plastic or vinyl for easy cleaning.

(2) *Therapeutic unit*
To an activity theory is added belief in therapy and rehabilitation. Staff are dominant, but provide for resident participation. Common statements are: 'you don't have to but I'd like you to join in'; 'it's good for you'; 'if you just sit, you'll lose the ability to walk'.

Developmental aspects are stressed, as with the horticultural model.

A blind eye is turned to disabilities and so success is judged in terms of accomplishments while in reality dependence may be increasing. The resident is consulted about admission and the opportunities are emphasised.

Creativity or personal fulfilment are important (though they may be unattainable to many) alongside tasks which residents are able to manage. Less emphasis is placed on the efficiency of the organisation.

There is consultation by senior staff with junior staff and residents; the head is 'head of home' and social work trained; staff do not wear uniforms and there is an overlap of jobs. Units are smaller, perhaps wing-type, with wings radiating from a central administrative block.

There is much greater use of normative control – the expectations of staff and other residents.

Residents are encouraged to be independent and to try to perform tasks, and the attempt is seen as valuable in itself; they are encouraged also to understand money, sort out change and go out to shop, though money may be given out centrally. Baths must take place regularly, but residents are stimulated to develop skills to bath themselves; similarly with cleaning arrangements. Staff encourage residents to participate in a 'treatment programme'. There is a choice of doctor, drugs are reduced and residents may hold drugs if staff agree. Residents influence menu and meal-times, but are encouraged to 'eat up'. They are given some choice of colour schemes and bring some furniture.

(3) *Retirement Community*
Common in America, unusual in Britain, the home offers a vision of a new life. Life continues to be active and purposeful while the resident makes decisions.

The old person decides to apply for admission. She plays a major role in appointing staff, with the consequence that the head is known as 'the manager'. Staff may wear uniforms, and have specialised jobs; they are seen more as employees. The buildings have good communal facilities including a bar, library and games rooms and residents have single rooms.

The next three types are based on disengagement theories.

(4) *Institution*
The essential elements here are withdrawal by residents from social activities, and minimal control of life-style. Indeed the withdrawal is involuntary, being forced on the resident by practices that exist within the institution. So the resident is prevented from participating in the life of the home and is given no responsibilities for her own life-style. Regimentation and block-treatment are combined with a staff belief that it is no longer appropriate for the resident to share in the hustle of life.

Some people may be formally admitted, decisions will be made by others and the resident told that 'it will be nice to let others cook/ clean, and so on', or 'it's time you gave up'. Doctors will be influential in this process.

There is a hierarchical system with the head known as 'warden'; staff are nurse trained and wear uniforms. As with the warehouse model, staff focus on the task to be accomplished rather than the needs of the resident. Buildings will reflect the wish to observe and control residents.

There are similarities with the 'nursing home' style in terms of minimal control by residents. The basic distinction is that in this model activity is seen as something that confuses. Residents do best when they are left in a settled routine; anything out of the ordinary will be detrimental. The apathy that accompanies this style is regarded as natural: 'it's sad for them but they have to accept that their useful life is over'.

(5) *Hotel*

The philosophy – that disengagement is natural – is similar to that above. However, residents are seen as people with influence. They must be consulted and their wishes taken account of. Residents and staff agree that a quiet life is best.

The resident is consulted about admission and encouraged because 'you will be free of all the chores'.

Staff influence over life-style remains great because staff control the resources. This is a particularly powerful situation when residents accept that they have few needs – relatives will be given their pension, and residents will be anxious to appear as gentle old people who fit in with all that is asked.

(6) *Flatlets*

This style reflects separate living-space for the old, but within that space a contented and happy existence. Restrictions and changes in life-style have been accepted and the resident has found a satisfactory *modus vivendi*. At admission, chosen by the resident, the resident acknowledges that former roles of parent, worker, club member have much less significance; therefore she will be happier in a situation where less is expected of her.

The final three models develop from a socio-environmental theory of ageing.

(7) *Home*

The word 'home' of the title is intended to convey the picture of the institution that endeavours 'to be just like home'. Here staff control is linked to a theory that allows differential explanation for individual residents. Staff acknowledge that individuals have different resources but they set the expectations for the group and for each resident. So one person may be expected to do more: 'what sort of life is that for someone who is as fit as she is?'. While another may be excused inactivity: 'well she's 93, you can't expect much'.

(8) *Hostel*
In this style staff set the rules of the establishment but within that framework residents are given freedom to select their own life-styles. So staff might say: 'we ask them what they want and fit in where we can'. When consulted about admission, prospective residents will be told: 'provided you fit in with the home, you'll be able to do what you want'.

(9) *Supportive unit*
Here resident dominance is combined with a socio-environmental theory of ageing. People are limited by resources and norms and how well they cope is dependent on how well resources and norms match. A major distinction from other styles of resident dominance is that residents may be physically dependent while making decisions about life-style.

Admission is requested by the resident who was aware that she would have greater choice of life-style in the old age home than in her own home. She would also be aware that staff would support her in her choice.

Residents play a major part in establishing the pattern of living; contracts making formal demands on staff may be drawn up. The weakness of the residents' position is that they may be a less cohesive group. But they have potential power to hire and dismiss staff. The head of the unit is known as 'the manager'; units may well be smaller, having a mixture of trained staff. It may be that fewer staff are employed or staff may change some of their functions.

The living style is controlled by the resident – with similar bounds to those that exist outside the home. Consideration must be given to fire risks and health hazards from neglect or incorrect medication. Otherwise residents are free to allow rooms to get dirty; to allow themselves to get dirty; they call the doctor when they wish; they have some choice of food, meal-times and they (or relatives) may cook some meals. Privacy is ensured by locks to doors. Residents are free to request staff help with tasks.

It is important to stress that the models are developed as a first stage in considering the link between events and attitudes and in opening up a discussion about the appropriate style for an old age establishment. Provisos need to be made in addition about the control of life-style variable.

'Control of life-style' is significant for several reasons. There is a long history to the feelings that residential institutions make people powerless. While it is necessary to consider rights for children, it is still more important that adults be given the maximum opportunity for making decisions. Studies of services for children which have used scales to measure attributes such as block treatment (King, Raynes and Tizard, 1971) have as a baseline that individual control of space or possessions is important.

King, Raynes and Tizard developed a scale – the Child Management Scale – which is designed to give a picture of the extent to which a unit is institutionally oriented or child-oriented. They pick out four areas – rigidity of routine, 'block-treatment', depersonalisation and social distance – and use questions related to these areas to give a total picture of an establishment.

'Rigidity of routine' is described as follows – 'Management practices are institutionally-orientated when they are inflexible from one day to the next, and from one inmate to another . . . ' – and includes as the first two questions:

(1) Do the children aged 5 years and over get up at the same time at week-ends as they do during the week?
(2) Do the children aged 5 years and over go to bed at the same time at week-ends as they do during the week?

In old age homes it is far more difficult at present to be sure of the components of good care. While there can be little justification for treating all of the residents in the same way, any particular resident of an old age home may choose an inflexible pattern of living and profit from going to bed and getting up at the same time.

'Block-treatment' refers to dealing with residents in batches, depersonalisation to providing no opportunities for personal possessions or privacy; both of these components provide useful ingredients for institutional analysis. However, 'social distance' again brings in a dilemma. 'Management practices are institutionally-orientated when there is a sharp separation between the staff and inmate worlds. This may be because separate areas of accommodation are kept for the exclusive use of staff, or because interaction between staff and children is limited to formal, and functionally specific, activities.' In an old age home social distance may be almost a basic human right, for residents may not wish to have intrusions made on their lives.

If it is accepted that maximum feasible control of life-style is a valid goal with the elderly it is important not to measure its attainment solely in terms of indicators which have prejudged what is the appropriate life-style. Therefore an incident, such as getting up or bathing at a regular time, may be an indication of either an inflexible regime which imposes this on a resident or an indication of a choice made by a resident and supported by the staff. The linking of 'control of life-style' and 'models of ageing' (which draws on attitudes and assumptions) allows a more appropriate examination of these issues.

The discussion of key factors in analysis of old age institutions will be picked up again in chapter 11 together with an examination of the distortion that can be created by measuring certain factors (such as control of life-style) and ignoring others (such as stability of staff and tenderness).

Chapter 3

PARTICIPANT OBSERVATION IN
OLD AGE HOMES

On one occasion at The Pines Mrs Draxton said to a care assistant: 'I don't love you any more.' There followed some discussion amongst other residents before the care assistant replied: 'I know what that's about – she had left some things out on her bed and we put them away for her, for her own good. Well Matron wouldn't have liked it.' Mrs Draxton retorted: 'Well, I'll know for the next ten years.'

Such an episode raises basic questions about research methods and interpretation. How reliable is the evidence? Did the observer affect the outcome? Would the same result be repeated in other comparable situations? What hypotheses explain this particular event? Which is the most likely of these explanations?

This book draws on material from a study of a single establishment. The dangers in such an approach have been documented by Tizard, Sinclair and Clarke (1975). They stress the need to look at factors that make one establishment different from another:

> [Our] approach highlights the differences which exist between the institutions at the same time as it makes it possible to evaluate their effects. By contrast, early research relied heavily on the single case study, so that it could only be generalised on the untested assumption that any one institution is an adequate representative of its fellows. This book tests that assumption and shows it to be false.

Thus it would be entirely inappropriate to draw on Mrs Draxton's interaction and to presume that there was a rift between all residents and staff at The Pines, and still more inaccurate to extend the conclusion to a general assumption that in old people's homes staff and residents fail to understand each other. However, in a situation where there is little idea of what are the right questions (or the key variables) the single episode may provide useful clues.

In fact, what is offered is a series of scenarios, or photographs, of a particular home. Provided that we remember the limitations of the photograph – a particular lens was used, the photo was taken from a particular angle, in a particular light, and so on – it is a useful way of capturing some aspects of an event. Similarly with this material – some pictures of a scene are presented but the limitations must not be forgotten. Hall *et al.* (1975) also consider that, given safeguards, the case study has value. In particular they suggest that it is 'a valuable means of conveying the immensity of the task confronting those who embark upon the journey from description to generalization in this terrain'. They add that such studies are 'suited to the "action" approach and to the exploration of the meanings actors attach to their behaviour in policy-making situations'.

PLANNING AND METHODS

Following detailed study of one establishment I hoped to gain some understanding of significant events and processes. Particular aspects were specified before going into the home – attitudes to ageing, admission processes and consequent changes in life-style, the formal and informal expectations of all involved in the home, a picture of daily life, choice and control, life satisfaction objectives of the home.

Attitude to ageing was one of the variables used to construct the typology of old age homes. Its significance is apparent from the way actions are influenced by beliefs or assumptions. For example, one resident, Mrs Hendon, stated that the home was a hotel and that she was there temporarily.

> I go out to work for a spinning company – well I don't go now, I'm out of work, getting on for 80. Sometimes I get miserable. Now I have got the house to myself I am well occupied, I don't get bored. I've always been one for getting up early; my daughter gets up between seven and eight. I have what I fancy for breakfast. If my husband has days off we go out to dinner.

Staff members assuming either that confused old people should be humoured or that they should be confronted with reality would treat Mrs Hendon differently. Questions about 'attitude to ageing' placed some of these assumptions in a broader framework. I asked: 'What is your picture of successful ageing? What sorts of things should old people do? Is it important to keep working? Do you look forward to or dread old age? A central aspect of the study was that the assumptions of different groups were examined: these included residents, staff, relatives and workers from the neighbourhood.

The second variable, *control of life-style*, differs from the more usual analytic idea of 'institutional control'. The distinction is necessary for two reasons. First, 'control of life-style' examines the situation from the point of view of the resident and charts the extent to which a resident has mastery of her own life. Secondly, since there is little known as to which situations are found to be most restricting by the old, it is necessary to start from a study of the types of control that can be exerted by residents. In addition ideas about institutional control have developed from work with children, and it is more essential for adults in residential homes to make their own decisions since they have done so for most of their lives. Mrs Williams said that sitting and waiting for a meal made her feel like a child at school. Whether it is right or wrong, children are more used to being managed in groups than are adults. When adults find themselves in comparable situations they recall their childhood dependency.

I selected some particular moments or happenings and used these as 'indicators' of life-style. These are listed below, together with some questions.

(1) *Money* Who holds pension books? What words are used to describe the pension (e.g., 'pocket money')? If given out by staff, where is it distributed (at office, in lounges, individual rooms)? Is money spent by staff on goods they decide are necessary? Who controls expenditure of group money such as 'comfort funds' or sums raised at special events?

(2) *Cleaning* Who decides the frequency, the time and the way in which the room is cleaned? Are residents allowed to leave the room in a muddle or dirty?

(3) *Daily programme* What choice do the residents have about the time when they get up or go to bed? Are events arranged for them? Are they expected to attend various functions including occupational therapy, communion? Do residents or others initiate visits, outings? Are residents and visitors free to come and go when they wish?

(4) *Bathing* Do staff or residents decide the frequency and the time of day for a bath? Do residents have any say in the way they are bathed? (Is it possible to choose between being left to lie in a bath on one's own for a few minutes or, if worried, having constant attendance?) Do any residents bath themselves? Do residents or staff select the clothes residents wear after their bath? Who decides which staff member will bath a resident?

(5) *Drugs and doctors* Do any residents hold their own drugs? How are drugs distributed? Is there any indication of over-medication, especially of confused or awkward residents? May residents choose their own doctors? Are residents seen in private by the doctor? Are the residents able to call a doctor or is this negotiated with staff?

(6) *Meals* Is there any choice of menu? Is there any flexibility in the time of meals? Are residents allowed to miss meals if they are in

the home? How are meals served? Are there serving dishes on each table or are meals served centrally? Are residents able to negotiate what they want? Is there any pressure to eat up or not to waste? Are residents allowed to cook anything? Are residents allowed to make drinks of tea or coffee for themselves or their visitors? Is there any choice as to where a resident may sit?

(7) *Individuals' rooms* Are residents allowed to decorate their rooms (paint the door, wallpaper or paint walls)? May pictures or ornaments be hung? What sort of furniture, if any, may be brought in? Are residents allowed to carpet their rooms? Do residents have a key to (a) the door, (b) a cupboard, or (c) a drawer in their room? May they put their name on the door? Is there a letterbox on the door? Are small possessions and ornaments allowed to be displayed or is it considered that they get in the way of cleaning?

The aspects for study listed earlier (p. 31) provide information which may be used to relate 'the various elements of the formal structures and processes of institutions to the informal life which operates within them' (Lambert, Bullock and Millham, 1970). However, the subsequent work of these authors at the Dartington Research Unit stresses also that their perspective tries 'to consider the dynamic implications of the individual's definition of his situation' (Millham, Bullock and Cherrett, 1975b).

So, for example, the interaction of Mrs Draxton and the care assistant cannot be understood by examining the goals of the establishment and the methods of social control. Mrs Draxton does not 'simply respond to social pressures in the manner of some robot', she evaluates her interaction with others and redefines her own position. For her this was often confusing and she felt she had a low position in the eyes of others.

Life satisfaction tests
There is no easy way of measuring happiness or someone's satisfaction with her life. In an interview a resident, Mrs Roberts, talked about life at The Pines.

It's a bit early to get up. My breath's bad in the morning. I do a bit, make the bed, wash, do some washing up. At nine-thirty I read the paper, look forward to that. I'd rather do without breakfast. Then some knitting, crochet and organising the football pontoon. All the days seem long. We used to get a young fellow with an electric organ, now he doesn't come. They used to enjoy it, have a sing-song. We need a public phone, we use the phone in the office. There used to be a phone in a booth in one of the lounges, it was in the wrong place, needs to be near the doors. I look forward to going to the pub. The food is very good here but there's no choice, you can't expect it, and they do change the menu. I sleep after lunch. I've got my own TV but don't get a good reception. I need an outdoor aerial. I've asked about it but I don't know what to do else. The lounge is too hot, I'd use my room more if the TV picture was better. Can't always watch what I want in the sitting room, I like sport. In the summer I go outside, in the winter stay in and watch TV. They're afraid of a mouthful of fresh air here.

How satisfied does she appear to be with her life? What extra information would a test provide?

Since 1949 there have been a variety of tests and scales developed to examine morale or life satisfaction. These have focused on the attitude that the individual holds towards herself and, as Gubrium points out, this is a significant determinant of a person's control of her own behaviour. Gubrium, in fact, sees morale as being dependent on a match between expectations being made of an individual and her resources to meet those expectations. However, at the conclusion of his work he attacks the picture of life satisfaction in as far as it is linked with 'the myth of the golden years'. He argues that:

the image of life satisfaction is built on a single conception of adjustment. To be adjusted in old age, it is implied, is to exhibit the following behaviour: (1) above all, to be 'happy', (2) to be altruistically involved with younger persons, (3) to maintain a 'busy' everyday life, and (4) to accept voluntarily the comparatively deprived social conditions that exist for many aged persons.

In effect this conservative approach expects old people to adjust to and be happy in situations that are demonstrably miserable and unsatisfactory.. Dissatisfaction would be a more healthy response to such conditions.

Provided it is not assumed that the life satisfaction index ought to indicate high satisfaction, the test is a useful measure of an individual's perception of her situation. The particular test used in this study was Life Satisfaction Index B (Neugarten *et al.*, 1961; see pp. 120–1 below for example of use in this study).

This test is a shortened version of Life Satisfaction Index A. The test has been criticised by Bigot (1974), amongst others, who considered that a particular selection of these questions provided a fuller picture. However Life Satisfaction Index B was used in this study because it employs a number of open-ended questions, as well as being designed so that it may be scored.

Both open-ended questions and scoring helped in understanding Mrs Roberts's view of her life. Although she appeared to be managing her life better than many residents since she was more active and lively, the Life Satisfaction Test showed her considerable dissatisfaction with her present life. In fact she scored 11 on the test and was below the average score for the home of 13.

Her responses to the first four questions clearly illustrate her feelings.

(1) *What are the best things about being the age you are now?*
It's a pity you have to get old. Why do you have to suffer? Go through a lot of aches and pains.

(2) *What do you think you will be doing five years from now?*
Kicking up the daisies.

(3) *What is the most important thing in your life right now?*
To get rid of my aches and pains.

(4) *How happy would you say you are right now compared with earlier periods of your life?*
Other periods were happier. Much of a muchness.

The test proved easy to use and the scoring range showed clear differences between residents. It was of value in testing out assumptions of contentment, as with Mrs Roberts, since some residents whom staff thought very happy scored low on the test. The other useful aspect was that the questions encouraged thoughtful reflection on the part of respondents.

THE STUDY AND ITS DEVELOPMENT

The particular home to be studied was selected by the local authority. The main areas of consideration were that the home should be one with a stable regime, that the head should be agreeable to the scheme and that the home should be geographically convenient for me to reach.

The Pines is a purpose-built thirty-six-bedded establishment with twenty-four single rooms and six double. It is near the town centre and, as important, near a main access road to the town. There are shops and a pub in the immediate vicinity.

The building has stairs and a central lift. The six sitting areas, accommodating between four and nine residents, are open-plan. Downstairs there is also a kitchen, dining room, small staff room and an office. Upstairs there is a laundry and a sewing room. The bathrooms are mostly on the top floor; there are several lavatories on both.

On my introductory visit one of the senior staff explained that the home had been opened seven years previously as the first of three new homes to replace an old institution. All of the first thirty-six residents were transferred on one afternoon in two hours. Three of the present

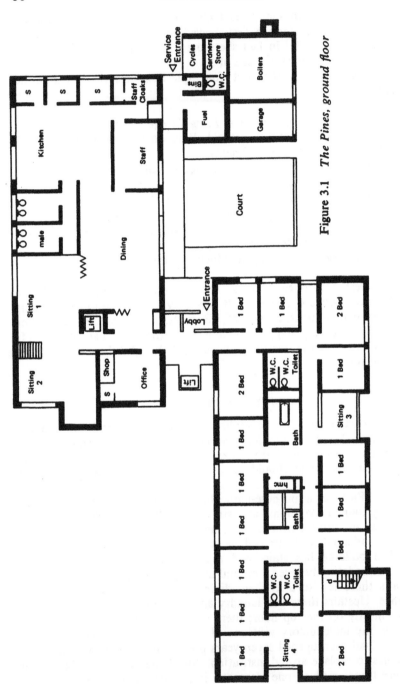

Figure 3.1 *The Pines, ground floor*

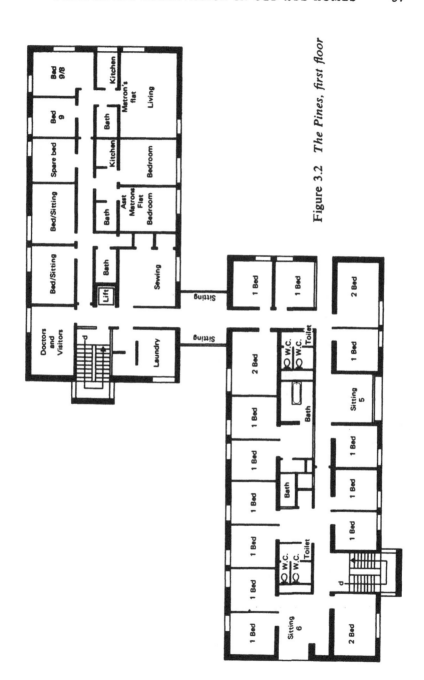

Figure 3.2 *The Pines, first floor*

six female care assistants had worked in the old establishment, as had one male care assistant. The matron and one of the assistant officers were appointed to open the home; staffing increases had led to the appointment of two other assistant matrons, one full-time, one part-time. The historical context is important because it is easy to present a picture of an organisation as static, whereas those within the organisation may be aware of considerable changes over time.

At the opening of the home a senior staff member had been told by the welfare officer 'It will take ten years to get rid of the institution atmosphere' and, when I spoke to her, the staff member thought that was right. The staff who had transferred to the new home had been concerned for their jobs and for the changes that might be demanded of them. One of the significant changes for the senior staff had been the progressive reduction in working hours and the introduction of set 'times on'. 'It is more like a supermarket now' was the comment because of the regular change in staff. Senior staff were no longer necessarily around at times of illness or death. 'I never thought it would come to this' said a senior staff member.

A synopsis of the study
The purpose behind this project was:

> To study a particular old people's home with the intention of making links between its practice and a typology of old people's homes worked out in advance, specifically to understand the attitudes to ageing of the people within the home, and interested parties outside, to see what relationships there are between attitudes to ageing and practice within a home.

The project covered eleven months and could be divided into three periods.

(1) *September–December.* At the start of this period in my research notes I used the word 'drift' to describe my involvement, with the idea of demonstrating being taken with the tide. At this time I needed to get to know people, to give clear messages about my purpose and to be around with different groups of people and at different times. In addition I began to look at the information available on various indicators (e.g. meal-times) so that I could relate The Pines to my typology. At the end of this time I met people who worked outside the home and developed an interview schedule for use with residents and a questionnaire to distribute to other groups.

(2) *January–March.* During this period I interviewed residents and produced and distributed the questionnaires which were given to staff, outside professionals and a few relatives.

(3) *April–July.* I started analysis of the questionnaires and produced reports for staff and outsiders and a summary report. Towards the end of this period I had the luxury of more free time in which I could take residents for walks or sit and chat. During the year I produced three newsletters for staff and residents.

Methods used

These were (*a*) participant observation, (*b*) interviews with residents (and a few staff), (*c*) a few written comments from staff and residents, (*d*) administration of life satisfaction tests to residents, (*e*) question-naires to staff, relatives of residents, field social workers, other interested professionals (health visitors, doctors, nurses), (*f*) studying available records such as staff rota, menus, logbooks.

(*a*) *Participant observation.* The observer is not neutral and therefore measures need to be taken to focus and structure the observation. A first step is to specify one's own values. Some of my comments before starting were:

> My picture of old age includes life having some purpose; the poten-tial for an old person to choose how he or she would live; the old being treated as responsible; some fear of increased dependence – especially physical disability (e.g. not being able to read), eneuresis, confusion. I find it hard to believe that sitting round and being bored is the result of real choice, nor do I believe in organised activities to anaesthetise and stop thinking. Neither forced inactivity nor forced activity can be right.
>
> Things that make me angry: staff being cruel, uncaring, laughing at or babying residents – and so creating the conditions they deplore; rigidity of routine; public living; boredom, loneliness, apathy of residents; lack of interest of staff; powerlessness of residents.
>
> Things I like: the possibility of privacy; concern expressed by gentleness; no bullying; the resident in control of the situation; enjoyment of life; death discussed and treated openly.

A second safeguard is to test findings against an established framework. (My framework was the table of models and the indicators.) While there are risks in participant observation it is often forgotten that there are risks in other methods. For example, even collecting statistics proceeds from a value assumption that such information is important.

Far outweighing the risks of participant observation, however, are the advantages – of understanding the meaning of a situation for the people involved, of discovering new perspectives, indeed, of finding that a new set of questions has to be examined.

Thus Miss Hutchins, a nearly blind resident, with severe walking difficulties, hobbled slowly back to the sitting room after lunch. A care assistant said 'Come on then, lift that right leg a bit' and the resident walked quietly by. She was regarded as a meek and contented person though often disoriented in space and time. In fact, having passed the care assistant she muttered: 'Does she think I do it on purpose? They'll find out when they are older.'

A second example illustrates the way a new area comes to be examined. I was sitting in the entrance hall before breakfast, while residents passed on their way to the tables. Mr Jepson came out of the lift and rested on his zimmer walking aid. He looked up at the slow-moving procession of people with sticks and zimmers. 'It's strange how it happens, you're all right one day.' This was the first pointer to the importance of considering adaptation to disability, as well as adaptation to residential living.

There is, of course, no way round the fact that the situation is altered by the presence of the observer. This must be acknowledged and the observer needs to use resources to minimise the effect, for example, by sitting outside a sitting area and recording movements, as well as sitting inside and joining in the conversation.

Another procedure is to record details of an incident and then get the differing explanations of people involved. Getting to know the observer over time will change the situation from one of guardedness to a situation where his presence, though noted, is not the most significant aspect in any interaction.

At the beginning I tried not to get too closely identified with any one group within the home. I joined senior staff for coffee-breaks, care assistants at lunch, went to each sitting area to meet residents. It is easy to forget the uncertainty of staff about what to do with me and the uncertainty of residents as to exactly what I was meant to be doing. A staff member recalled at the end of the study how fed up she had been when asked 'You'll take Mr Clough with you, won't you?' on my first afternoon. A resident at lunch was anxious that I needed help from the staff to find out what to do. Another explained my presence to a visitor by 'Oh, he's from college', which obviously explains everything! Similarly I was concerned about the impression I was making and the best way to record events.

I joined in as a staff member serving meals, taking round the drinks trolley, helping residents to stand and walk, making beds and, occasionally bathing. In this period I made sure that I was present early in the morning and in evenings and at night-time, as well as during the day.

It was more difficult to observe staff without my presence modifying behaviour. For example, I joined a care assistant bathing a resident and found the care assistant talking to me, when normally she would have conversed with the resident. Even following a member of staff round had its difficulties. I followed a care assistant round as she woke residents with a cup of tea. From one room the man said 'Come on, then'. 'No, not this morning' was the reply. And to me she said: 'They're funny some of them. He likes a kiss in the morning.' Presumably had I not been there, he would have had it.

Situations where I was not so conspicuously an observer provided more typical material. Serving in the dining hall it was easy to be working and also to be aware of the interaction of other people. An advantage of open planning for me was that I could be in one room and hear the conversation in another!

Another early problem was to communicate ideas to staff and residents since there were no staff meetings and no residents' meetings. The production of a news-sheet solved this and the first one of these aroused much more discussion than I had expected. Residents said: 'I read it and put it away to read again'; 'I like to see something that's independent'; 'I like reading things like that, very interesting'. There were comments too from staff – a cook said that it was very good but that I would never really know what the job was about until I had cleared up a mess after someone.

I used this and subsequent news-sheets to let people know what I was doing, and to propose ideas, such as residents writing about a day in their life.

Another difficulty with being an observer is to provide clear information about one's purpose. As I went round with one of the senior staff I had constantly to correct the picture that was being presented. 'Mr Clough is here to check, to find out . . . ' Not surprisingly one person responded with 'You won't find anything to report on here'. I was aware from my introductory visit of the need for a precise form of words, which was 'to find out what it's like for people living and working in an old people's home'. Several months later, when I began interviewing residents, one resident was overheard to advise another not to take part on the grounds (imaginary!) that I was a Jehovah's Witness out to convert people.

Detailed notes were kept on incidents and conversation during each day. These were used both to record and to raise questions to follow up in other ways.

(b) *Interviews.* The interviews with residents (see Appendix 2) were not tape-recorded. I had neither the resources to get all the interviews typed up nor the time to cope with the mass of paperwork involved. I made detailed notes, recording actual phrases where possible. This was helped by (1) the somewhat slower speech of many residents and (2) the fact that I paused to complete notes.

The full interview lasted between one hour and one-and-a-half hours. Nearly all of those residents interviewed were able to concentrate for this length of time, which surprised me. The interviews were spread over a period of several weeks. Only one person asked me when she was going to be seen and several, from comments fed back to staff, found it a difficult experience. One woman felt giddy after forty-five minutes, and never wanted to complete the interview; another stated that old people should not be harassed, that she should have been asked in advance (she had been but had forgotten), that she intended to consult her lawyer (a frequent riposte of hers). Needless to say that interview finished very quickly!

During the interview period there were thirty-nine people in residence (including one holiday visitor). Of thirty-nine possible interviewees, twenty-six were interviewed, three were judged too ill by staff, one was unable to speak, following a stroke and nine, for a variety of reasons, did not wish to be interviewed. This last figure, 23 per cent of the total available, is higher than I should have liked. I was aware of the residents' dependency and anxious to allow them a real choice. The only people I was prepared to persuade were two who said they had nothing 'good enough' to say. Of the nine who refused interviews, four had lived in the old workhouse. (There were nine residents from this workhouse – considering that one of these had also failed to complete the interview, 56 per cent of the ex-workhouse residents refused or did not complete interviews; three were very withdrawn, holding minimal conversations within the home; two felt they did not want to recall past problems.) Another person who refused was deaf and would not wear a deaf aid. I thought it would be too much for her, while the remaining three did not give precise reasons.

Interviews were held in residents' rooms except for one that finished in a pub since it was time for the interviewee's regular Guinness.

The interview schedule which I developed proved of more value in some parts than others. Multiple-choice questions were difficult to use. For example with question 21 about the aims of old age homes, I wanted interviewees to select one of four statements as the most important, or add others of their own. In fact hardness of hearing coupled with some difficulty in remembering all the items made it impossible to answer without considerable development of the question by me. This leads me to question the appropriateness of multiple-choice questions with old people and, indeed, the reliability of evidence drawn from such questions.

The questions that aroused the greatest response were those that asked for descriptions, in particular questions 11, 14 and 18: 'Do you remember how you came to think about admission to a home?', 'Can you tell me what happened when you first arrived?' (followed by prompts such as 'Did you come by car?'), and 'Can you tell me what you usually do during a day?' (with prompts such as 'Do you take long to get dressed?'). Questions that asked for direct answers sometimes had to be explained at great length and too many possible leads were then given about answering the question.

(c) *Written comments.* The few comments received from staff or residents contained some useful viewpoints. While this idea of diary writing is worth pursuing it is probable that it will only gain little response.

(d) *Life satisfaction tests.* These proved useful and have already been discussed (pp. 35–5 above).

(e) *Questionnaires.* Three different questionnaires were produced for staff (see Appendix 1), for interested outsiders and for relatives. Each had a different set of questions but had in common a series of statements about old age with which respondents were asked to agree or disagree.

Ten out of twelve staff completed questionnaires. Information was confidential, for staff were asked only to fill in their job descriptions, not their names. Matron and the assistant matrons used the term 'senior staff'.

I hoped to get information about: the perceived goals of the establishment; the satisfactions and dissatisfactions of the job; attitudes to old age and specifically to activity as a model of old age; those seen as the most popular, most unpopular and happiest residents; attitudes towards residential care; the importance attached to various tasks; possible changes in the running of the home.

Two sets of questions failed to get the desired response. In the first (questions 11 and 12) I asked which residents staff got on with best and which residents staff found least pleasant. These brought out a strong commitment to an often-stated policy within the home of 'no favourites'. While I knew this policy existed, I had not seen my question as being at variance with it. Three of four senior staff made specific comments: 'In my position I do not have favourites, they are all treated alike'; 'It is the policy of the home not to have favourites'; 'Definitely no favourites'. Those care attendants who made specific points stressed that 'I get on with everybody', 'Mostly get on with all of them', 'Everybody, including staff, can have an off day', 'Each has good and bad points'.

Only one person listed the people with whom she got on best, and she said that she could not say anyone was unpleasant. The question would have been better phrased in terms such as 'If you had a few minutes to spare to whom would you go and chat?', or 'Whom would you avoid if you could?'.

From the second set I hoped to get a picture of individuals' perceptions of the way they would age. However, the actual questions (25 and

26), 'Which resident do you think you will be like when older?' and 'Which resident would you wish to be like when older?', probably seemed too flippant.

The second set of questionnaires was sent to 'interested outsiders'. Those approached were given a stamped addressed envelope, and this was followed up by a further letter requesting return of the form. I spoke on separate occasions to social services department staff, a GP practice lunch-time meeting and the physician and ward staff from the geriatric hospital.

Thirty-two questionnaires were returned: twelve from social services department staff, seven from GPs and a physician, four from health visitors, three from nurses at a geriatric hospital, three from 'friends' of the home, two from district nurses and one from a county councillor.

Six relatives completed a third questionnaire. There was no easy way of communicating with relatives. Several residents were concerned not to worry their relatives with the questionnaire, even at times when the relative had already indicated that she would complete the form.

(f) Records. Immediate records of menus, drugs, or of residents' ages and dates of admission were available. However, there was very little written of any length. Official visitors recorded their visits and made little comment, and the senior staff quarterly comments to the social services committee were primarily about numbers, the weather and outside events. The sparsity of information is itself a comment on the style of running the home.

The final stage. Research workers frequently collect a mass of information from a wide range of people. The information is usually confidential and gives to the research workers immense power. Researchers must find appropriate ways of sharing that information and should avoid producing a report after they have left an establishment, when it may not be possible for them to discuss the findings.

I had agreed to feed back my ideas in the third phase of the study, April to July. The production of the reports emphasised my committed stance. While my task was to share the perceptions of the home, gained from my own observations from interviews and questionnaires, the selection of the material was bound to result from my bias. Therefore my standpoint before going into the home (p. 39 above) needs to be considered alongside any subsequent findings. Thus I was not neutral simply by being a researcher.

Three reports were produced during the study period. The first, for staff, was based primarily on staff responses to questionnaires but included some details from interviews with residents and my own observation; residents received a synopsis of this in the form of an extended newsletter. The second report was for outsiders and brought together perceptions of different people about admission and residential living. The third report, primarily for senior staff from the home and the department, highlighted some of the main findings while adding riders to earlier documents.

The first report had the most impact. I reported the feelings of staff and residents, described some events and offered explanations of events. My aim was to raise questions about practice but not to offer solutions. It was important to separate tasks since it was not for me but for others, the homes adviser and senior staff, to implement change if that was thought appropriate.

My objectives in producing the report were: (1) to produce a report that would get read – not too long, avoiding jargon, safeguarding confidentiality; (2) to build up a desire for change by shaking the complacency of staff; (3) to stress those areas which concern staff, for example, 'staff should not gossip'; (4) to take account of factors stressed by Rothman *et al.* (1976) which promote the preconditions for change; (5) to promote discussion amongst staff so that some norms might be exposed and questioned; (6) to stress specific areas of concern – (*a*) the admission process, particularly the loneliness, and the uncertainty at nights, (*b*) the powerlessness and dependence of residents, (*c*) the open discussion of residents and staff.

The production of the report and the reactions to it contain many of the central issues of the research. In fact it brought to a sudden halt the automatic acceptance of my presence within the home for I had been careful to avoid feeding back my impressions at an earlier stage.

For me it brought out the basic tensions between understanding what was happening and my lurking wish, which surfaced occasionally in various progress reports, to stop some things happening and produce change. The need for clarity of task pushed me towards the job of explanation of events but the frustration of not making statements about ways changes could take place was real, though I knew that if change was to occur it had to arise from and be implemented by those with responsibility for the establishment. In fact to be involved directly as a change agent it would be essential to be invited in for that purpose; change from the approach adopted in this study would be slower but might lead to a re-examination of methods in residential homes generally.

The report aroused mixed feelings among the staff. One care assistant was quoted as saying that she would never speak to me again. A senior staff member was described as 'unhappy or sad about it'. She was thought to be hurt because the residents had said the things they did. It was thought also that she saw nothing positive in the report. To me she said she felt that she might as well give up the work. Three members of staff regarded it as valuable, with material for discussion.

So I had to face the impact of my report but also the question, rightly raised by staff, as to the objectivity of the report. The incidents quoted were real and the statistics accurate, but they were selected to highlight certain aspects of residential living. Such selection is inevitable but it must take account of issues that concern other staff and residents as well as those noted by the researcher.

Two staff meetings held to discuss the report were chaired by the homes adviser. The reports – and meetings to discuss them – were the last of the formal aspects of the project.

Personal summary
The challenges of the first part of the study were about presenting myself and the details of method. So I was aware of the importance of confidentiality – and of saying repeatedly that I did not pass on information – of not becoming identified with one group, and of having a simple statement of purpose which also was repeated frequently. In terms of method I had to plan my time, work out a reliable form of note-taking and cover as many sources as possible – for example, circulars from county hall, minutes of Friends' meetings, lists of drugs, information on files – as well as discuss these items with staff. In fact it was a period of structure.

The structure continued into the period when developing the interview schedule and questionnaire. After that the structure was clear at particular moments – for instance, interviews, developing reports – but there was an increasing amount of informal involvement. In sitting with a group of residents or staff I was less concerned to steer the conversation to particular topics since I already had a mass of information on these.

One aspect that I was aware of from the beginning was that my presence might be intrusive. There is no doubt that residential institutions have been ready targets for research because of the captive situation of the resident. Therefore it is all the more necessary for the researcher to be sensitive to the feelings of residents.

A more complex problem arose when I started to produce progress notes on the research. To structure these notes I used the headings taken from the original analysis – control of life-style, with its various indicators, and attitude to ageing. The picture that emerged seemed a little distorted for, on reading the report, one person commented: 'I hope that I never have to go into a home then.' I felt that there were elements of the home that I had failed to capture. One possibility is that my involvement was already making it difficult for me to face up to the negative aspects of the home.

Another possibility needs careful consideration. This is that the variables selected are important, but on their own do not portray a full picture. Aspects such as security, dependability and continuity need far greater emphasis than they were given in this study. While they may be less easy to measure, such additional variables will demonstrate other aspects of life in a home. The gap was partly covered by looking for a range of opinion, from residents, staff and outsiders, and by examining the goals of the organisation but, nevertheless, failure to broaden the analysis will only perpetuate 'the myth of the evil institution'.

Another key area for me was the growing awareness that attitudes in old age are linked not only to personality characteristics but to other factors, in particular mobility and health.

An adult who has coped successfully with a variety of stress and change may still find it difficult to cope with whatever happens in old age. So the challenge is not only to theories that rate personality as the key variable to survival in old age; it is also to one's perception of one's own life when older. If I were so restricted in mobility that even getting to the lavatory became a wearisome effort, would I be as bitter as some of the residents. Certainly there were several who felt life was pointless or that they had been dealt a cruel hand by fate.

It should be stressed that the bitterness frequently had nothing to do with residential living – it had developed because life had become too much of a burden. I tried to reflect these feelings in a poem I wrote two months after starting the project. It expresses the futility or despair shown by a few residents and it illustrates also the effects on the observer. It is significant that the despair of the few may have a more marked effect on staff or visitors than the contentedness of others.

The poem starts from some typical comments of staff or residents.

'You've got your memories' – Yes, memories bring
Roses in December and children in old age.
But are we destined to become nothing but an album of past snaps?
'It's something to do' and 'it fills in time',
So, you knit and you knit and you knit,
Items that nobody wants.
There are feet that will not listen,
There are eyes that do not lead;
Bladders that are punctured and that leak.
Bodywork that's dented, hinges rusted up
Machines that can't be mended, only left to creak.
'Keep going', 'Keep trying', 'Keep moving' –
But 'For what?' I want to scream.

Two residents in particular, a man and a woman, faced a struggle, either with themselves or their legs, to keep walking, even with the aid of zimmer frames. It is in an area such as this that the perspectives of different groups are valuable. A geriatrician felt such a person must be kept mobile; staff differed in their response to the statement 'I can't walk today', depending on their own inclinations or that of senior staff. Some would wheel the resident in a chair to the dining hall; others would encourage the resident to walk one way and wheel him back in the chair; others would get the resident to walk both ways. Residents, watching a scene like this, would comment that it was for the resident's own good or think staff were being too strict. Underlying a lot of what was being said was a feeling, only occasionally made explicit, that a resident who lost all mobility would be transferred to a geriatric hospital.

Faced with the tears of the resident leaning heavily on the zimmer, the supposed struggle of the observer for objectivity is given up. (Perhaps it is put in abeyance since the preceding paragraph shows that in fact different perceptions of the situation were recorded.) While not opposing the wishes of staff, I would try to pre-empt such situations, or, if the individual was going to have to walk because staff said so, then ensure that I helped her as gently as possible. There remains no way of escape from the fact that the observer has no authority to change existing practices. It may be possible, when performing staff tasks oneself, to fulfil them in a different way. It would be pleasant also to be able to record that the result of the research was significant changes in practice, but it is too early to tell.

Some other points need mentioning. This was the first time I had seen the body of someone who had died; and I remember touching the body in the quiet of a small bedroom and talking with a staff member, for whom also this was her first sight of death.

From the interviews I became aware that residents needed help to get some things accomplished. There was a man who wanted to write but whose right hand was useless after a stroke; a woman who could not get adequate reception for her portable TV; several people frustrated by the life they were leading.

In the period after the production of the report I made it clear to staff that I was available to help in ways they wished and increasingly took an initiative in proposing things that I could do. So I took residents in wheelchairs round the town, to the pub and out in the garden; I took residents out with another member of staff for drives and a picnic; I helped the man already mentioned to learn to use a typewriter so that he could write letters; I took a discussion group of four residents when we talked about religion. All in all, I enjoyed the luxury of more time to sit and chat and do what I wanted.

The project came to an end with a special lunch. The home had won a 'Jubilee' turkey from *Woman's Own*, staff and residents sat down to eat it – at separate tables but for the first time staff were eating with the residents – the wine flowed freely and then I found myself feeling quite emotional during some speeches, and it all ended with hilarity as I was given the bumps.

A visitor quoted back at me a passage from my report to outsiders that spoke of the dominant picture of the home as 'a rather pleasant ordered calm'. 'Peace at last' said a senior staff member about my departure!

Chapter 4

———◆———

COMPARATIVE BACKGROUND INFORMATION

The thirty-six residents at The Pines comprise a small percentage of the total number of elderly people who live in residential homes, about 150,000. This group is itself only a small proportion, about 2 per cent, of the total number of people aged over 75 in the population. A brief discussion of such trends in the population and in residential institutions is included so that later information about The Pines may be placed in a broader context.

OLD PEOPLE IN BRITAIN

The old (taken to be over 65, unless otherwise stated) are increasing both in number and as a proportion of the total society (see Figure 4.1). In this age-group the very old have increased at a faster rate than the younger and there are substantially more old women than men. In addition, women are more likely to be in need of services to help them since at all ages they are more dependent, less mobile and more likely to live alone. The very old are more likely to live in worse housing and to be poorer than other old people.

The growth in numbers of the old is apparent from the fact that

in 1901 there were 1½ million people aged 65 or more in a population of just over 37 million. In 1971 the respective figures were 7·1 million and 54 million. In percentage terms the over-65s had increased threefold from 4·0 per cent to 13·3 per cent, while the population was not quite half as much again in the same period. (Jeffrys, 1977)

Those aged 65 and over now constitute 14 per cent of the population of England and Wales. Two-thirds of this pensioner population are between 65 and 74 years and one-third are over 74 years. This latter group is composed of twice as many women as men and is where most of the real frailty is concentrated. Proportionately these older 'olds' are increasing at a faster rate. The women, mostly widows, are more dependent than the men who mostly have wives still alive. The male robustness reflects the fact that they are a group who have survived the critical middle-age years for men (35–55) when heart disease and cancer are major killers.

Figure 4.1 *Population aged 65 and over, England and Wales, 1951 and 1977*

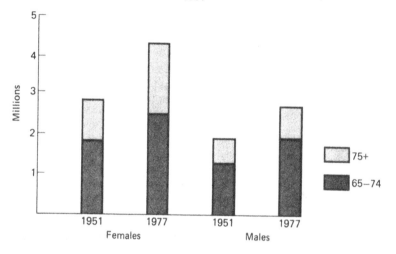

In 1977 there were 824,000 men aged over 75, while there were over twice as many women: 1,780,900.

The trend for those aged over 75, and even more significantly for those aged over 85, to become an increasingly large proportion of all old people is expected to continue to 2001. Thus by 2001 women aged over 85 will be 11 per cent of all elderly women (cf. 1951: 4·8 per cent) and those aged over 75 will be 48 per cent of all elderly women (cf. 1951: 34 per cent).

The importance of these figures is demonstrated by comparing them with age- and sex-groups of those in need of services. It is women over 75, and in particular over 85, who make disproportionate demands for services.

Thirty per cent of elderly people live alone. Hunt (1978) shows that nearly 80 per cent of all those who live alone are women, and over 35 per cent are women aged 75 or more. Not surprisingly the chances of living alone increase with age, though women are more likely to live alone at any age. This is partly explained by the fact that men are more likely to be living with a younger spouse than women and that women live longer. Thus at 85 or over nearly 31 per cent of men are still living with their wives in a separate household. By contrast only 4·5 per cent of women over 85 are living with a spouse in a separate household. Sixty-six per cent of women aged 75 or over are widowed or divorced.

Hunt's study also shows that the 65–74 age-group are not much more disadvantaged physically than the age-group immediately beneath them. Indeed, people of 65–74 tend not to consider themselves old However, the small percentage of this group who need services is still a significant total, for the group comprises about two-thirds of all elderly.

According to Hunt, 4.5 per cent of the elderly population were bed-fast or housebound and this increased to 20·6 per cent of the over-85 group. It is important to note that women at all ages were less mobile

Figure 4.2 *Age composition of local authority residential homes, England and Wales, 1966 and 1973. These figures include a small number who were supported by local authorities in voluntary or private homes*

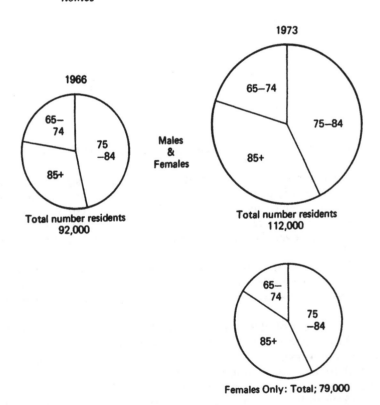

than men. Power (1979) shows a significant drop in women's mobility between the 75–79 and 80–84 age-groups. For example, 61·7 per cent of women aged 75–79 could move freely, whereas only 41·9 per cent of the 80–84 group were able to do this.

Impaired mobility is a major cause of dependence on others. For those aged 75 and older, 7 per cent of men and 12 per cent of women cannot leave home unless assisted. A second major cause of dependence is confusion, although there is disagreement as to its meaning. Meacher (1972) argues that much confused behaviour arises from problems of social adjustment while others contend confusion is brought about by physical factors in the brain. Whatever the cause, the reality is that the confused elderly may need people in constant attendance to watch over them.

RESIDENTIAL INSTITUTIONS

Of the 151,000 residents of old age homes in 1977, 30 per cent (46,000) lived in voluntary or private homes. Staff often state that their task has changed considerably – on admission residents are more handicapped, more confused than they used to be. It is said that residential homes are being asked to run as nursing homes or mini geriatric wards without the nursing resources of either of those establishments. How far is this an accurate reflection of the present state of residential homes?

(1) *Age of residents*
Older residents are a growing proportion of those in old people's homes (see Figure 4.2). The major increase in numbers, even over a short seven-year period, has been for women over 75, in particular for women over 85.

(2) *Dependence of residents*
It is much more difficult to chart increased frailty because measurements are far more reliant on the subjective interpretations of staff. This point is borne out in several places in the Census of Residential Accommodation. Some examples of the statements made about ways of collecting data are:

> The information provided by the homes relied upon the judgement and memory of those completing the forms and must therefore be treated with some caution. Respondents were asked to give details of the condition of the residents over the two weeks preceding the census and this meant that they should have accurate and up to date information about every resident. Opinions may have differed on definition of terms . . . (DHSS, 1975)

This point is emphasised again in relation to mental condition described as 'the least objective of the dependency measurements, as it is easily affected by observer bias; a particular resident is likely to be judged relative to the overall condition of residents in this particular home'. Finally, the development of measures of dependency is described as the most important area for improvement.

Nevertheless the survey does provide some information. Four factors were examined: continence, degree of mobility, self care and mental condition (see Table 4.1). Women, as would be expected, were less able to care for themselves than men. There were variations in levels of dependence between authorities (London boroughs had far higher proportions of dependent residents), but they do illustrate the large numbers of residents who are continent, able to walk around the home, and can feed themselves. Even with vague terminology like 'mental confusion' over half were judged mentally alert.

Table 4.1   *The abilities of female residents from local authority homes*

Percentage of all female residents judged to be:	
Continent	69
Able to walk unaided	44
Able to feed self	96
Mentally alert	52

Source: DHSS, 1975.

These figures, although dating back to 1970, are the most reliable available of the national scene. Hughes and Wilkin (1980) compare evidence from a range of sources. However, nearly all the material quoted is based on local survey and the DHSS (1975) survey is the only one which examines figures for England and Wales.

There is some possibility of comparison between Townsend (1962), whose fieldwork was carried out between 1957 and 1961, and the DHSS survey. Townsend found that 52 per cent of new residents needed little or no help to live in their own home; 61 per cent of women and 83 per cent of men were able to walk outside the building; 14 per cent were incontinent, 54 per cent needed help in bathing and 19 per cent in dressing. The DHSS (1975) survey shows an increase in incontinence and a dramatic fall in numbers able to bath themselves. The latter may be partly explained by the clear policy of most authorities that residents are to be supervised at bath-times which is likely to lead to undermining of residents' ability. Even allowing for this the change is significant, and particularly so in the light of the time that is given in staff hours to bathing residents. There are few residents in residential homes today who would need little or no help to live in their own homes.

A survey in East Sussex of applicants to residential homes examined capacity looking at nine areas concerned with personal care, physical health and mental health: 9 per cent had no incapacity and a further 16 per cent incapacity in only one area.

Table 4.2   *Category of residents in dependency areas, Cheshire*

	Mobility	Personal care	Mental state	Behavioural problems
Residents needing little or no attention	82	63	68	70
Residents needing attention	18	37	32	30
Total	100	100	100	100

In Cheshire a survey examined the dependency of residents (see Table 4.2). Four areas were specified: mobility, personal care, mental state and behavioural problems. Residents were then divided into one of two categories: those needing little or no attention and those who needed attention (Kimbell and Townsend, 1974). This survey is useful because it followed up this material by examining how far residents had clusters of problems. Forty-three per cent of residents were shown to have problems in none of these areas – in other words they needed little or no attention to carry out functions in any of the four categories.

Brought together, these pieces of information suggest that residents are more dependent than was found by Townsend but that a substantial proportion of residents remains only minimally dependent. This is reinforced by the DHSS (1975) survey which found that nearly half of the residents required little personal assistance from the staff. The finding is extremely important in considering staffing and styles of living within the home.

(3) *Marital status of residents*

However, it is useful to consider the other factors that may have contributed to admission since incapacity does not account for the total number of admissions. Age of residents has already been examined and it is clear that the very old are more likely to need residential care. Marital status is not mentioned by the DHSS or East Sussex surveys but the Cheshire survey shows the high proportion of widowed and single amongst the residents (Kimbell and Townsend, 1974). Ninety per cent of all residents were single or widowed, with 64 per cent of these being widowed (see Table 4.3).

Table 4.3   *Marital status of residents, Cheshire*

	Single	Married	Widowed	Divorced	No reply	Total
Percentage of residents	26	5	64	3	1	100

The proportion of single people is higher than for the population as a whole which is readily explained since without children they have a smaller network of relations on whom to call. Incidentally it should be noted that the number of children available to care for their parents has fallen with the fall in the birth rate. Evans (1977) shows that the number of potentially dutiful children available to support their parents fell by 19 per cent between 1951 and 1971.

(4) *Previous residence*

There is considerable consistency between the DHSS (1975) survey and the Cheshire study. Of those in local authority homes, 30 per cent were admitted from hospital (DHSS, 1975). The full figures are given in Table 4.4.

Table 4.4   *Previous accommodation of residents in local authority homes*

Previous accommodation	Percentage of residents in each category
Sheltered housing	2
Other housing – living alone	24
Other housing – living with others	21
Hotel/boarding house or lodging	3
Another residential home	19
Hospital	30
No settled residence	1
Total	100

The large number – 19 per cent – who were admitted from other residential homes is largely accounted for by the closing of large, old institutions and the opening of new homes, though a smaller number would comprise those who were being transferred for other reasons – to move them nearer their former home or relatives, to cope with particular dependent residents in a more appropriate setting. The more surprising figure is that nearly one-third of all admissions came from hospitals. This indicates both the degree of handicap and the way in which a major break in the living situation appears to make the past pattern of caring an impossibility. Relatives may realise the effect on their own families of caring for a parent when the stress is removed. Of course this does not make clear the previous residence of those who go into hospital. Townsend (1962) suggests that 50 per cent of all admissions were from people who were living alone – a much higher figure than for the elderly population as a whole. Harris comes to similar conclusions. She found that 47 per cent of all residents had been living alone and 41 per cent living with others. A further 69 per cent had lived in a hotel or boarding house and another 6 per cent with a spouse. The under-representation of the married is again demonstrated, together with the over-representation of those living alone.

(5) Reasons for admission

Inevitably it is difficult to explain why people enter residential homes. A combination of factors so often exists that there is some distortion in listing the prime reasons. It has already been shown that incapacity on its own does not explain either application or admission to residential homes, although residents are more dependent than comparable age-groups in the general population (Harris, 1968).

Townsend's (1962) analysis has received substantial confirmation. Acknowledging that homes now take older and more dependent residents, there is widespread acceptance of additional factors that need consideration. Townsend listed the following:

Lack of close relatives and friends
Loss of supporting relatives
Separation from family and community
Consequences of isolation
Difficulties of living with the family
Homelessness
Housing conditions
Financial insecurity
Lack of domiciliary services

Perhaps the biggest change has been in the growth of domiciliary services. Many new residents have had considerable support from home helps and meals on wheels which contrasts with the picture painted by Townsend.

Harris has a much briefer section on reasons for admission. She states incapacity for self-care as the basic reason, often following illness at home or in hospital. Those who do not want to be a burden on children are another large group, and this may be associated with family friction. She cites 7 per cent of residents as wanting company – a positive reason for admission that stands out from the usual picture of lack of resources. Finally she mentions a small group with financial problems and a large group for whom housing is a major problem. This includes both poor facilities and homelessness.

The East Sussex survey found the two major reasons for admission were family problems and physical illness. It is interesting that those who stated physical illness were less incapacitated than any other group; it may be significant that 90 per cent of those who gave this reason were living alone and they may have felt an exaggerated sense of infirmity (East Sussex, 1975). The writers conclude that:

> there is evidence that factors such as homelessness, poor housing, isolation and loneliness and family stress were important and therefore that provision of services to combat these problems could have reduced admissions. These conclusions appear to follow fairly closely those of Townsend made over twenty years ago.

In a study of field social work Goldberg (1970) found only ten people who went into residential homes. Clearly this is too small for any firm conclusions but it may be significant that prior to admission six out of ten had said they were often or sometimes lonely and four were rated as discontented or openly unhappy by the assessor. This was a higher proportion than for those who remained in their own homes. Her concluding comment is: 'Thus in this tiny group it looks as though social reasons, both situational (housing) and personal, rather than incapacity in itself, are associated with entering a home.'

(6) Planning and choice

Admissions result, then, from a combination of stress factors. There is a hint from Harris that a small percentage of people wanted to go into a home for the company they would find but most writers pinpoint problem areas. This method of analysis seems appropriate for it matches the way most residents respond to questions about admission and illustrates the normal pathway to a residential home. A conglomeration of problems results in a crisis; the crisis leads to re-evaluation of the situation with the consequence of admission to a home. While for many admission may be *the best choice of living arrangement that is available*, it is almost never part of a planned change of life in old age.

There are exceptions to this. Some people do plan for a stage of life when they will need more support and then they have a choice available. They may get a friend, relative, or companion to live in; they may move to a smaller, more convenient house; some people plan to move to a private hotel; others buy flats in housing associations where support is available and a few plan to move to a voluntary or private home for the old. There is virtually no planning for entry to a local authority home because the resources are too scarce and are used to meet whatever is assessed as the greatest need. The possibility of admission at an earlier age to a voluntary or private home makes planning more realistic.

(7) Building programmes

Poor housing conditions are often a factor in necessitating residential care. The standard of housing provided by residential homes has shown a dramatic improvement. Indeed, one of the most consistent and expensive trends in social services must be the building of new homes for the old since 1948, but in particular since 1958. The major change has been in building over a thousand new medium-sized homes in England and Wales. In 1959 there were 443 medium-sized homes; *by 1973 there were 1,806*, a growth of over fourfold. In 1959 42 per cent of residents were living in large homes (over seventy places) with only 31 per cent living in medium-sized homes (thirty-five to seventy places). By 1973 77 per cent of residents were living in medium-sized homes and only 12 per cent in large homes. The change is all the more amazing when it is remembered that total numbers of residents grew from 60,900 to 100,400.

These medium-sized homes accommodated far more residents in single bedrooms – in 1970 30 per cent of all residents in local authority homes had single bedrooms with a further 32 per cent in double rooms. A DHSS Building Note in 1973 suggested that a maximum of one bedroom in nine should be a double room and all the rest be single rooms. This has not been achieved, but significant progress has been made. A further point in the Note is that there should be one WC for every four beds, and in 1970 only 30 per cent of homes met these requirements.

There is a basic tension between raising standards in existing homes and building new homes, and this is emphasised by the large sums of money that have to be spent to keep abreast of changes in fire regulations.

Staffing

Between 1966 and 1973 the number of residents increased by 39 per cent. In the same period the number of senior staff (matrons, wardens and their deputies) increased by 54 per cent and the number of care assistants by 69 per cent. These increases are in whole-time equivalents, not gross numbers, so they are real increases. This means that there has been an increase in real terms in the numbers of staff (full-time or equivalents) that has exceeded the increase in the numbers of residents. However, it must be noted that the average number of hours worked per week has decreased in the same period so there has been little improvement in the number of hours of staff time available per resident. The ratio of senior and care staff to residents was 1:4·7 in local authority homes for the elderly. Interestingly voluntary homes had a slightly worse ratio of 1:5·3, but this was compensated for by more domestic staff, and they had less dependent residents.

There has been little increase in the numbers of qualified staff between 1960 and 1970. In 1970 83 per cent of local authority senior and care staff held no qualifications. Nearly 90 per cent of those qualified held a nursing qualification. Over half of those with non-nursing qualifications had attended only a fourteen-week course. So there were very few with any social work qualification.

Figure 4.3 *Population of The Pines, Somerset, and all local authority residential homes, 1966, 1973 and 1977*

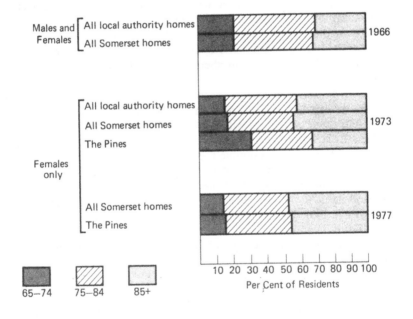

THE PINES AND SOMERSET OLD AGE HOMES

The proportion of older residents in Somerset old age homes has increased in line with the national average (see Figure 4.3).

Table 4.5 shows the previous residence of those admitted to Somerset residential homes in 1976–7. It is apparent that more people in this sample were admitted from hospital than in the DHSS survey in 1970 (38·5 per cent compared with 30 per cent).

Table 4.5   *Previous accommodation of those admitted to Somerset homes, 1976–7*

Previous accommodation	Percentage of residents in each category
Sheltered housing	7·0
Other housing – living alone	17·7
Other housing – not living alone	7·0
Friends, relatives	19·3
Hospital: general	14·7
geriatric	18·3
psychiatric	5·5
Local authority home	6·1
Other home	2·8
Other address	1·5

Dependency trends in Somerset can be compared for 1970 and 1978 (Somerset County Council, 1978). The numbers of residents who were substantially dependent remained the same, at 15 per cent of all residents. However, there was an increase in those moderately dependent from 40 to 50 per cent of all residents. Significantly most of this shift in overall dependency levels is attributable to residents aged 85 years or over. It is this age-group which has experienced the greatest shift from 'minimally' to 'moderately' dependent.

The differing dates of available figures have not allowed a direct comparison between the Somerset and the national figures on dependency. However, it is useful to see the figures for Somerset alone (Table 4.6).

Table 4.6   *Somerset long-stay residents' self-care abilities, 1978*

	Dressing	Washing hands and face	Bathing	Use of WC or commode	Combing/ brushing hair	Feeding self
Alone – no difficulty (percentage)	54	62	10	69	70	84

My period of study at The Pines was a year before this survey. Similar patterns were apparent at The Pines, though in a small home the figures in any box might change markedly from week to week.

Thus in so far as comparison is possible between all local authority homes and those in Somerset, the trends appear remarkably similar.

Chapter 5

———◆———

GOING INTO A HOME

INTRODUCTION

There are, then, an increasing proportion of women over 85 who are residents in homes but such trends do not explain why some 85-year-old women apply for and are admitted to residential homes and others do not. The most comprehensive study examining this is one by Tobin and Lieberman (1976) in America. After a thorough review of other findings and a well-constructed research programme that was detailed in method and looked for changes over time, they emerged with the following conclusions. 'There is little reason to doubt that a wide array of types of people apply to and become residents of homes for the aged . . .'

They consider three variables to be important in explaining the reasons for entering a home: 'personal deteriorative changes in the older person, the inability or unwillingness of responsible others to offer the care that they or the respondent perceive to be required and the inability of the current system of services to assure independent living'.

Of particular importance is their finding 'that factors other than personality types must be used to explain why some older people and not others apply for admission to residential homes'. This is vividly illustrated by their case studies which show *over time* how individuals responded to changed circumstances. Events, such as death of a significant person or physical deterioration, might change people's attitude to life.

It has already been stated that an individual rarely plans in advance to enter a local authority residential home. The result of changed circumstances – of particular clusterings of events – is admission to a residential home. In this process the old person rarely initiates discussions with the social services department, the body responsible for running the home. Townsend (1962) writes: 'It was somewhat surprising to find that comparatively few of the new residents in our sample had acted on their own behalf and many of the local welfare agencies which might have been expected to play an important role in fact played a small one.' He found that it was the doctor, whether in hospital or general practice, who frequently played a significant first step. He continues: 'The old people did not take the same view as others of the conditions in which they were living and of the attractions of residential care. Doctors, for example, often told them that it was not in their best interests to remain in insanitary houses, and relatives argued that they should not live alone any longer without adequate help.'

THE INFLUENCES OF THE DOCTOR AND SOCIAL WORKER ON ADMISSIONS

The doctor had been a significant person in seventeen of twenty-six admissions in the present study. This figure would certainly be higher if information were more precise: for example, some of the ex-institution residents did not remember who had been involved in arrangements, while one confused woman did not think she was in a home at all. In eleven of twenty-six admissions the doctor is reported as having *instigated* the process.

> The doctor asked me a year before I came in. 'Not yet', I said.

> The doctor said I had to give up. I had mixed feelings.

> The doctor said, 'You can't carry on like that'. It was a bit of a shock.

> The doctor suggested it. My daughter would have had a breakdown.

The doctor is the professional who comes into contact with the largest number of old people. There may well be others, home helps, district nurses, social workers, who have more intensive contact with *certain* of the elderly, but the doctor has the wider range of contacts. He also has more status than the other group and people *as patients* have become used to accepting recommendations. The doctor has also become used to *making* recommendations. Nevertheless the frequency with which the doctors had suggested admission to residents, and the authority given to their pronouncements, surprised me.

When social workers were already in contact with the person, as was the case with two women who were registered blind, the social worker was as likely to be chosen for help as the doctor. Relatives mentioned consultation with a social worker as much as with a doctor, presumably because social workers are more involved with detailed planning of admission. When consulted, social workers were less likely than a doctor to suggest admission to a residential home.

It is sometimes assumed that doctors are unwilling to supervise old people who are at risk in their own homes and that they too readily suggest the old go into a residential home. Social workers, on the other hand, give over-riding consideration to independence when perhaps the struggle of daily living *restricts* independence. Doctors, who see more of the struggles of the very frail old, in this study took a more negative attitude to old age than other groups (see p. 170 below), seeing it as more dreary, less of an opportunity to do new things, more boring and more depressing. There may be more times when doctors appropriately question whether the old should stay in their own homes than social workers may acknowledge.

> The doctor advised me to go into a home. I talked to my family who didn't want to hear of it. They didn't want to see my side. I had a home help three mornings from eight-thirty to ten a.m. but then had to manage on my own. I did the cleaning and the fires; lugging coal was a problem. I could manage the meals, and did the washing up. Some days I felt I didn't know how to carry on. My family didn't want to part with me. Brother would come and see me most mornings, would bring in a bucket of coal. There was no bathroom; the toilet was downstairs.

In this situation Mrs Richardson was living on her own, housing was restrictive, she received considerable support from home helps and had regular contact with her family. Nevertheless, 'some days I felt I didn't know how to carry on'. There is no easy solution to her problem. Since she lived in the country rehousing would involve a move away from her family and it is impractical to consider a greater range of domiciliary services. For her the best alternative was a residential home. Any choice had severe limitations and this will need to be remembered in later sections when the restrictions of residential living are examined. These must be balanced against the restrictions of other styles of living.

It would be useful to have more detailed information than was available from this study about the actual knowledge of all parties (doctors, social workers, relatives, prospective residents) about particular homes. How far are major life-decisions for the elderly made on casual recommendations from others?

While the great demand for local authority homes makes choice *between* homes difficult, the choice between staying in one's own home and moving to a residential home should be made with detailed knowledge. For those who plan to pay for residential accommodation there is more choice, but I suspect many decisions are still made on casual hearsay. Two themes are worth pursuing further: the *routes* by which different groups of the elderly approach residential homes and the ways in which people may find out about styles of living in old people's homes.

The perceptions of different people about strengths and weaknesses of residential living (see pp. 173–6 below) are also important influences on the decisions of the old. The evidence in Chapter 11, though from only a very small sample, suggests that doctors were less aware of the psychological aspects of entering a residential home than were social workers.

REASONS FOR ADMISSION

It was shown earlier that ten interviewees had lived with others before admission. These living arrangements broke down for a variety of reasons, of which the most significant was hospitalisation either of the old person or some crucial person in the care-system. In two cases the caring daughter went into hospital, in another two the old person. The spell in hospital would seem to have made a tenuous situation impossible. Harris (1968) makes a similar point.

> Quite often this stage [of not being able to look after oneself] is reached immediately after a spell of illness, treated either at home or in hospital. Doctors in hospital often recommend a residential place before discharge where an elderly person lives on his or her own, particularly when housing conditions are bad. A number of the elderly go into residential accommodation because their doctors recommend it as they might fall when on their own, or because they are advised against being on their own at nights.

However, these points would seem to apply more to an individual living alone. The significant fact in relation to the care-system is that the problems related to the illness are coupled with an opportunity to demand a change. Hospitalisation is conspicuous and can become the event that leads to change.

Of the remainder who lived with others: one person's daughter was said to be on the verge of a breakdown; the 73-year-old resident housekeeper of another needed a rest; in another case the caring daughter was moving away; while one woman felt she was in the way of the grandchildren; and one woman who was living with a friend of a similar age found she could no longer do enough herself to make the situation viable.

Those living alone gave the following as reasons for admission: six spoke of problems of managing the house 'It was getting beyond me, I couldn't get upstairs'; 'I kept on till I couldn't cope – I was spoiling cooking pans'; two mentioned poor housing, in particular dampness; one could not manage following an accident; two were thought too confused to continue managing (social work report); one was considered 'at risk' with respect to health (social work report).

Several residents stressed that they preferred a residential home to living with children because they did not want to be a burden, nor did they wish to feel restricted.

I wasn't getting any better; I was relying on my family so much and they had to lead their own lives.

I've only got a daughter. I didn't want to be any burden.

I made up my mind too quickly. I had my daughter to think about.

One woman described why she stopped living with a relative:

I lived with my husband's grand-daughter for nine years. She was very kind, had two children. I used to get in their way; it wasn't pleasant for the children or the parents. 'Don't get in Nan's way' she used to say.

I lived with my youngest son for twelve months. 'I don't want to interfere in your life; I'd rather go in a home' I said.

I had thought I might live with my son. They had only three bedrooms and one large sitting room downstairs. The children needed the beds. My daughter-in-law likes meeting people and going out – she goes out to work all day. My youngest son's marriage had broken up, my daughter only had a flat. I didn't want to go to the children if I was able to go somewhere else; I don't want to be a burden.

I couldn't go to my son. They are both out at work. Young couples have things all special. I wouldn't go there in any case – my daughter-in-law is very particular – she has got everything all new. I'd feel all on pins about knocking things over, marking the carpet.

There are two different strands in the reasons given for not being with a family. One strand acknowledges that the old person may be in the way of the family and risk being a nuisance, while the second stresses the wish not to be a burden and leads to an emphasis that the decision was that of the resident not of the family. Thus Mrs Smith emphasised that her family wished her to stay in her own home, as did Mrs Williams and Mrs Richardson. The fact that these three were all living alone prior to admission may be significant.

Tobin and Lieberman (1976) contend that the 'resident-to-be cannot afford to be rejected because the home has been determined to be the best, if not the only, solution available. To handle the rage and to maintain self-esteem, the resident-to-be usually emphasizes that the decision to apply to the institution was wholly his own.' They suggest that for some people this may be a reasonable mechanism for coping with anger and fear.

However, their proposition does presume that most old people have this fear of rejection. Twenty-six per cent of a group they interviewed on the waiting list for admission to homes introduced the issue of rejection when discussing changes in relationships. The difficulty is that, unless the fear of rejection can be demonstrated from other sources, there is a danger of assuming that all those who state that they themselves decided to enter a home are employing defence mechanisms.

An important dimension that was mentioned earlier is the part played by the professional workers in influencing decisions. Therefore it is essential to know any differences between groups of workers about reasons for admission and the purpose of residential homes.

In this study those working with the elderly in the town were sent questionnaires. The opinions about reasons for admission are shown by answers to two questions which distinguished between the main reasons that necessitated admission and factors that changed a viable situation into one that necessitated admission.

Two major sets of reasons for admission were given: (1) the inability of the old person to cope and (2) an inadequate support-system. Twenty-one people mentioned the inability of the individual to manage. This included 'frailty', 'self-neglect', 'danger to self', though many used the phrase 'unable to cope' which presumably meant an inability to complete the daily tasks of living. Most groups of professionals mentioned this as a reason.

An inadequate support-system was noted by nineteen people. Here comments included relatives or neighbours being unable to cope, friction or breakdown between some members of the household, death of a spouse – all of these suggested a breakdown in an existing support-system. The absence of any support-system was a reason given by six people. Significantly health visitors and social workers concerned with social situations all gave considerable weight to an inadequate support-system, whereas doctors did not. The nearest comment by a doctor was 'no care or supervision at home'.

Poor health was a third area mentioned. This included immobility, mental and physical disability, malnutrition, illness and recovery from illness, and was mentioned by eleven people from all professional groups.

Isolation was mentioned in five replies. This covered lack of contact with others, lack of interest in life and loneliness. Other reasons given included accommodation, the preference of the individual and no other alternative.

The inadequacy of the support-system was given even greater weight when considering reasons that made a situation intolerable. Twenty-eight responses mentioned insufficient support or support that had broken down through death, moving away, or changing expectations of the 'care-takers'. The circumstances detailed about the individual old person are similar to responses to an earlier question, though deteriorating health and illness or accident were given very much greater emphasis. Surprisingly doctors rarely mentioned health problems as the factor that changed a viable situation into one that was not; it was health visitors, followed by social workers, who saw these as most significant.

In fact there seem two basic patterns. In one situation the elderly person goes to live with a son or daughter and the stress of the physical caring or emotional involvement become too great, a fact which is often brought home when the situation is temporarily changed through hospital admission.

In the second set of circumstances, an inability, or an unwarranted struggle, to complete basic household tasks leads to application to a residential establishment. The professional groups have a similar picture of the first pattern to those involved, but attach much less weight to the decreasing mobility of the elderly than do the elderly themselves.

OPINIONS AS TO SUITABLE AND UNSUITABLE RESIDENTS

It is important also to find out the characteristics of those who are seen as suitable or unsuitable candidates for residential homes, since it has already been shown how influential is the professional in steering people towards residential homes. Respondents claimed that they would *discourage*:

(1) Those able to care for themselves (ten responses). People who were coping adequately or were fit enough to stay active were mentioned under this heading.

(2) Those seen as independent (eight responses). 'Independence' was cited frequently, for example, 'those who were not lonely and valued independence'. A stronger statement was 'those with sufficient backbone to go it alone'.

(3) Those with unsuitable characteristics (seven responses). This included both people 'who would not mix well' and those regarded as difficult, awkward, or anti-social.

(4) Those with adequate support (seven responses). This group comprised those cared for by family, or other helpers such as neighbours or home helps.

(5) Those seen as too sick (four responses). This was used to indicate those too sick to be in a residential home, but it was difficult to define the boundary.

Other responses included 'those who could afford private homes who would not fit into a local authority home', 'those expecting a five star hotel'.

The picture of those seen as suitable for a residential home is far less clear. It indicates the lonely, those at severe risk, those with deteriorating health, those unable to care for themselves, the dependent and those without support. A large number (nineteen responses) mentioned one of these last three categories but the responses do indicate wide differences of understanding about the need to enter a home. For example, some thought a residential home was needed for those unable to care for themselves (a reply which would fit the perception of the old about reasons for admission); others coupled this with lack of support, while a further group added the word 'dependent'. While the responses do not make clear whether dependence is viewed in physical or emotional terms, the high rating given in the earlier question to those with 'backbone' staying out suggests that dependence is viewed in personality terms and negatively. The single word used most commonly in this answer was *lonely* – a clear statement that respondents would encourage the lonely to enter a residential home.

In effect the combination of factors that lead to admission has been illustrated. Residents are likely to be unable to look after themselves *and* to be lonely, or psychologically dependent, or without support. The different perceptions about the suitability of applicants are crucial because most residents had not considered admission before it was suggested to them. Since places in residential homes are a scarce resource some sort of rationing is inevitable. One aspect of that rationing is the influence of the professional worker but the discussion above has shown how haphazard that influence is. In considering which people should be encouraged to enter residential homes there was a very wide spread of answers though some clustering of views around the lonely and the immobile was apparent. This emphasises the dilemma between providing residential homes for those who will enjoy and benefit from them or those who could be said to 'need' residential accommodation, because they are at risk. If the first option is taken the anti-social or awkward are excluded, if the second these same people are included because they are 'in need of' a place in a residential home. While some respondents would consider the awkward or anti-social for residential homes, most would not. Different professions gave different answers.

ALLOCATION

Doctors stressed that they would discourage the fit, the independent, the self-sufficient, and would encourage those who were frail, forgetful, had decreasing mobility and those with poor support-systems. Probably because they were farther removed from management responsibilities they gave less attention than social workers to excluding those with unsuitable characteristics, nor did they consider placing those who would benefit from residential living.

Two aspects must be separated out. The first is the process which leads to application, the second is the way in which decisions are made about allocating places. In the first stage doctors have been shown to have significant influence, and the opinions of professionals as to who ought to go into a home are important. While doctors may influence significantly which people apply for residential care, it is the social services department that allocates vacancies. The local area team of social workers discussed at a meeting held with the writer the way allocations were made. A health and mobility scale had been used in the past to assess priorities for admission. Recently so many applicants had maximum points on the scale that it no longer discriminated effectively. For permanent admission they excluded those who were frequently incontinent, those unable to move around even with a walking aid and the mentally confused where this was likely to lead to a serious management problem. They gave priority to a person living on her own.

The pressures placed on the area team were considerable and show the marked contrast with most other residential provision under social services' control. While there is a shortage of places for any sort of residential home the demand for allocation comes from other professionals – for example, in the case of an unruly child from the school, from other social workers. With the elderly, the social services' department is subject to considerable pressure from relatives, doctors and even the elderly themselves. The local newspaper is scanned and the announcement of a death at an old people's home is followed by phone calls requesting that a particular individual be allocated the place. In addition individual social workers will be pressing the cases of particular clients.

The social workers in this team stressed the right of individuals to decide their own style of living even if it did not seem satisfactory to the social worker. They would uphold this principle in the face of their own doubts and pressure from neighbours or relatives. However, they would not face the threat of medical resources being pulled out, although they would endeavour to get a second opinion from the community physician.

This shows some of the factors considered by one area team of social workers. Other studies (East Sussex County Council, 1975) have shown that different divisions within one authority may have different methods of assessing whether an elderly client requires residential care. 'The amount and depth of information required to be provided by social workers varied considerably and so did the informal unwritten criteria applied.'

There have been attempts to standardise procedures within an authority. One such (Davies and Duncan, 1975) drew up minimal criteria for admission and a system of weighting applications. The establishment of minimal criteria (which include the wish of the elderly person to go into a residential home) demands that domiciliary services have been considered and that assessment is structured around certain headings. The priority groupings list six sets of social circumstances (housing, tension in household, at risk, disabled, mental disturbance, hospital) and gives four gradings of priority in each situation.

To return to the particular situation of this study, the process of application involved the applicant being interviewed by a social worker, and seeing a booklet produced by the local authority which attempts to answer some of the questions people may have about residential homes. Social workers felt the booklet was more help to relatives than to the elderly themselves.

MOVING IN – RUSHED DECISIONS AND LOSS OF POSSESSIONS

Except with urgent admissions the prospective resident has the opportunity of getting to know the home through a short stay or day care. Of twenty-six interviewees, five had been transferred from the old institution. Of the remaining twenty-one, seven remembered holiday visits, two had paid short afternoon visits, four stated that they did not want a trial because they knew the home, eight offered no information about this.

There was no correlation between residents who were most satisfied with current life-style (as shown by the life satisfaction index) and prior visiting to the home. What did emerge is that several people knew of the home from visiting friends, from coffee mornings, from singing in a visiting choir. So it is useful to consider ways in which the local community may get to know a home. Though a short visit is better than none at all, its unsatisfactory nature is shown by one resident who thought after the visit that she was to have a little flat on her own.

The extent to which a resident felt that she had influenced the decision to come into a home was closely related to life satisfaction scores. Those who stated they had decided to come in, often ignoring the wishes of their families that they stayed out, were more likely to be satisfied than those who came from care-systems that had broken down. This fits with Tobin and Lieberman's findings discussed earlier, though it does not assume such choice to be the result of a defence mechanism. In particular those who felt the decision had been made *for* them were likely to have low satisfaction scores. A man was unable to remember anything about coming in: 'See my daughter' he said – and he still hoped, totally unrealistically, to return home.

'I wanted to be independent, I don't know why I came in, I don't know why she [her daughter] got me in' said a woman, and this situation illustrated the pressure that may be applied, particularly to rush a decision. 'My daughter spoke to the social worker about it. "I've got the social worker coming in, what do you think about going into a home?" she said. It was a shock to me, I only had about a fortnight to decide.'

For others the pressure related to having to settle affairs too quickly, even after making the decision to go on to a waiting list for admission. Inevitably vacancies could not be planned but a typical response was 'when it came, it was sudden'. Interviewees described asking for more time and a staff member commented that most people take a long time to plan moving home to a new area whereas the elderly are expected to settle everything in a few days.

An extreme example is that of a woman on a fortnight's holiday visit to see if she liked the home. At the end of a week a death occurred in the home and it was decided to offer the vacancy to the holiday resident.

Her account of the incident is interesting.

Last May [eight months before] I had a fall. The doctor said 'Wouldn't you like to go into a home?' I didn't think anything more about it until just before Christmas [only one month before the interview]. Then a gentleman came to see me, he might have been from the housing, he took notes. He said that there was a bungalow or flat going empty. 'No, if I give up my home, I'll go to The Pines', I said.

Then a social worker came, the week before Christmas, and brought a card to say the dates [for holiday visits]. Then she came last night to say there was a room vacant, but I'd have to share. I got Matron to show me the room – it was rather small, I'd want to bring my own commode. What room is there to put things in? The social worker said I couldn't bring in much, so I'll leave it till I go and see. She said if I didn't take this opportunity there would be a wait. I wanted to come in before the winter but this is rather sudden.

She decided to take the offer of a place and was asked to take up residence the following Monday, six days after the first discussion. She was able to get this put back a week. There had only been about five weeks from the first serious discussion of admission to a home with a social worker. Clearly the administrative need to maintain high occupancy rates may be at variance with the needs of the elderly to have time to adjust to changed situations and time to make decisions.

The uncertainty of this resident about what she could bring in was common and several people wished they had brought in more. Other comments were:

I didn't know what to bring in. She told me, the welfare person, I could take a table or rug, could take an ottoman. I sold lots of things privately.

My daughter said 'Oh you don't want to have a lot of stuff'.

I took what I wanted. Brought my work box. The chest and carpet I bought since. Didn't want to bring in anything else, wanted to forget. I didn't want to be cluttered up, I get around better. I put my photos away. (A blind woman)

The dominant picture prospective residents appear to have had was that it was reasonable to bring in a commode and one or two small items. Some had not even understood this. There are six double rooms in the home and a new resident always shares a double room. This means that there is not much space for anything other than a commode and small items. Added to this it is made clear to residents that domestic staff like a tidy room without too much clutter around.

Others discovered that, when they moved into a single room, things for which they then had room had been given away.

'I gave away a lot of things that I wish I hadn't – lots of little things. I didn't know you could put in your own furniture.'

The rooms of two residents were a contrast. One decided to bring in a lot of things and got rid of those she didn't want; another was where a woman was unable to sell her house and therefore was able to go back to collect other things she wanted. Her room was a great contrast to every other one. It was cluttered up with bits of furniture, ornaments and a large sewing machine. A senior staff member said: 'She moves the furniture around and has it in her own individual style. The girls [domestics and care assistants] don't like it but I think if she can't get in it to sleep, that's her problem.'

Finally, two observations suggest that given active encouragement some more reticent residents might hang things up. In both cases the rooms were spartan with nothing around. One man showed me treasures of his in the wardrobe – photos of his parents' marriage – and described some fretwork and a mirror that had been stored upstairs and he'd never had up. This was similar to an experience when the room of a man who was leaving for hospital was being cleared up. He had nothing of his own around. Now from drawers and the wardrobe there turned up old photos of the man, young and handsome in the army, and an intricate woven sampler presented by his firm and wishing him well on retirement. Several staff members commented how easy it was to see only the present person, a shell of a man constantly wet and dirty, and to forget that he had been someone with a real past.

It is comparatively easy to remedy this by giving time to hanging up pictures. However the problem with furniture is far more complicated. Ideally residents need time to adjust to their new life-style before disposing of possessions. Modern purpose-built homes have little space for storage, and families, if not the resident, are anxious to tidy up the house the resident is leaving. Some social workers (at a meeting with the author) wondered whether it might be possible to find anywhere else to store furniture.

FIRST IMPRESSIONS

The following extracts give a picture of the memories of residents about the first few days.

Three people remembered coming from the old institution.

I didn't like the thought of going to the institution. I had heard so much about it, we used to call it the union. Had to go because there was nowhere else to go. The food was nice when we came here, had more meat.

I liked it coming here. A man came and showed me up to my room, a nice young fellow. The WVS brought our luggage, it was like a railway station. A good job we came here, nobody to interfere with us. It's nicer, happier, more at home.

I didn't want to come here. The other place was more comfortable, warmer and no draughts. You need doors here. There were no men there. The cooking is marvellous here, atrocious there.

This is a palace compared to that. People were happy there, heartbroken to leave [though she went on to say how much better the move was].

Others had come from their own home or hospital.

I had a good idea of what to expect, nothing was different from what I knew.

The welfare brought me. I came just in time for lunch. I have been in a good many places, I soon fell in.

I was excited about coming in. Surprised to see such a wonderful place. People were treated better than I expected. A social worker brought me in with my luggage. Matron met me and took me up to my room, an attendant unpacked and put everything away.

They greeted me and I felt pleased with the way I was greeted. Took me upstairs with my case. I didn't mind sharing a room because I felt there was someone to guide me with the lift. Brought me back down and I had a meal at dinner time . . . others kept me in conversation; I felt it wasn't too bad. The Pines felt like a home. The difference from your own home is not working any more.

The most important thing was feeling comfortable – nothing to worry about; able to rest; done my duty; surprised at such a place.

Another talked about the people – their moans and groans.

It's a different atmosphere. Mrs X is boss of the show. I had been in for a visit but when I came in it was sudden. I think a lot about what I left behind – little treasures, saving old-fashioned things, magazines, a favourite chair, a knife and cup, not a plastic mug; I use my own mug a lot. I miss the life around my home – everyone was jolly.

It's living with other people, not your home. You have to have what food is given; to make life decent you have to swallow so much.

It was not as hard for me as for some people, I was used to institutions. Had to be sure stuff was marked. The cooking is all right but it's not like home. I miss the salt, though sometimes I don't.

I miss the phone, my own possessions, miss the friends from home, the control of the TV.

I miss my independence. I didn't like it for three months till I got into the rhythm. Very handy, rather like it now – terrific things to get used to. I was used to deciding things for myself – cleaning, sewing when I wanted. I'd been in the army, used to discipline – the feeding arrangements didn't upset me. Living with other people is difficult, I can't describe it.

I came in June. It was a Monday morning, raining. It's nice with friends all round now. I used to clean my bedroom, make bed, cook the dinner. I miss not having enough to do, but got used to it.

I came in at tea-time, went straight into the dining hall. My son went straight off. Knew nobody. Felt all up to here [her throat] but got over it. The hardest thing was being waited on – led to the table, toilet and bedroom [she is blind]. I'm very independent and I like to do things for myself. They are kind and I ought to be grateful. I've got a placid nature – always done things for myself, I don't know other people's feelings – the different things people have to endure . . . The most difficult thing is not being able to go out for walks on my own. I miss the outdoors and gardening. I used to be up at eight and get the housework done by ten so that I could get out in the garden.

I miss my garden, had two nice lawns, grew rose trees [and she talked about a busy life with clubs and meetings, making 800 Easter cakes for a sale, and how she had wanted to cut herself off from all these things on coming into The Pines].

I came in an ambulance, was car-sick. I was shown my room, had one by myself to start with. It was difficult but I had been in hospital before. The people were most difficult to get used to – all were very friendly. At home it is quiet, no next-door neighbour. I lived next to the farm, I missed the noises of that for getting up, the cows going for milking.

Matron came and greeted me. I thought it was all very nice. I couldn't sleep for two or three nights. It was better than I thought. I remembered the old workhouse.

It is apparent that some residents arrived close to a meal-time and therefore went along to the dining hall soon after arrival. One had enjoyed this because she was 'kept in conversation'. However, it may well be difficult as an early experience for many people. A similar point is made in a recent review of residential care (Personal Social Services Council, 1977): 'Above all, he should not be led into a full sitting room and left to cope on his own.'

Two people talked about feeling lonely or not sleeping at night and staff comments on how this could be altered are discussed later. The essential part is to separate the aspects that cannot be modified – missing the noises of the farm – from those that could be handled differently, such as information about possessions.

The admission process appeared to me a crucial and neglected part of the way residents learnt to behave in a new setting. In the report which I produced for staff I drew attention to some points.

Several interesting things emerge:

(1) Residents often said they couldn't remember what happened when they came in. But when I asked who brought them and whom they met from the home they remembered a lot. In particular they remembered talking to a senior staff member, going to their rooms, going into the sitting room and their first meal. Therefore what happens on the first day is very important.
(2) The difficulty of being in a strange place at night-time. Loneliness and strangeness are most apparent then. For some residents the nights remain times of loneliness and pain.
(3) The little residents remember of anyone talking about what they could bring into the home. They had been told they could bring in a commode but others had left behind ornaments that they wished they had brought with them.

   Some had been able to collect these later; in other cases they had gone. 'I wonder what happened to my radio. I'd like that now' said someone. The concern about doing the right thing was so great that many people never brought in things they wished they had.

(4) From my observation of the admission of a holiday visitor: he arrived with the social worker, had a brief discussion with a senior staff member outside the office, was shown up to his room. Meanwhile the social worker came into the office, handed over his pension book, talked to staff members, said that he wanted his pocket money but would spend it if he had it. She left. Later a care attendant came into the office: 'I've unpacked his case and brought down these tablets.' What struck me was that initiative or responsibility was taken away at so early a stage. First, the social worker dominated the early discussion outside the office, she handed in his pension book, she said 'perhaps he shouldn't have his money'; the care attendant brought down the tablets.

To me this is an important example of the way responsibility is removed from residents. I believe incidents like this admission process are part of the reason for the apathy that nearly everyone seems to dislike. The comment of one of the residents – 'I took it as it came, resigned to doing what was expected of me' – is an example of what people expect to find.

(5) Those residents who were most satisfied were usually those who thought they had played a major part in making the decision to come in.

(6) The important point is that the first impressions lead on to fixed attitudes. In the example above other people (the social worker and staff) decided what would happen to the new resident – and so a resident gets used to a situation where other people make decisions for him.

Social workers who accompanied old people into residential homes were aware of the way the group of residents dominated proceedings at an early stage. They would tell a new resident not to put a bag down on a particular chair: 'That won't be her chair, she won't be sitting there.' Similarly an individual's picture of life in the home would vary according to which sitting area she went to. People had had very different experiences in one sitting area on holiday and then in a different sitting area next time they came in.

Staff felt that it was important to be hospitable to the new resident, and it is apparent from several comments that senior staff members succeeded in conveying their interest. 'Matron came and greeted me', more than one resident said. Some staff members suggested that taking a case and unpacking it is the sort of hospitality that one would show to a guest. 'How else do you show that they are welcome?' asked someone.

Nevertheless, the example of the holiday visitor illustrates a type of hospitality that leads to dependence. There is no reason why an admission scheme should not foster independence and convey warmth, if that is what is desired. Other examples of socialisation into set patterns of behaviour, for instance, keeping the room tidy, will be discussed later.

Chapter 6

———◆———

DAILY LIFE FOR RESIDENTS IN
THE PINES

The style of life of residents at The Pines is portrayed in this chapter through the eyes of myself as participant observer and of residents. A comparison can be made with the staff view in Chapter 9. Both the staff's and residents' viewpoints will have similarities to and differences from other establishments.

It is difficult to capture the key elements of life in a residential home. Discussing this problem, a geriatrician referred to trace elements in plants – elements which are present only in minute quantities, are difficult to analyse but are essential to the well-being of the plant. Hopefully some of these trace elements that make up the sound, sight, smell and feel of life at The Pines are captured in what follows.

A TYPICAL DAY

About 6.30 a.m. residents who will need a lot of help with dressing are woken up. The remainder will hear a knock on their door between 6.45 and 7.00 and the care assistant will bring in a cup of tea. Some residents are already awake – 'You're late this morning'; others slowly wake up. At 7.30 the care assistant does a second round and collects up the cups. One man says he doesn't feel well enough to get up. A woman asks for her red and black dress from the sewing room. Somebody else wants another blanket.

There is a bit more noise and bustle. Some people are sitting waiting to be helped with the next stage of dressing; others are persuaded to start getting up. One resident who has become highly dependent is left sleeping in her room.

8.00: Some residents move downstairs and sit in a sitting area till breakfast. Others go straight to the tables. The vacuum cleaner is going – 'We have to get used to that music' says a resident. There is a succession of greetings between staff and residents as different people meet. Residents greet each other more quietly.

The corridor from the lift is crowded with slow-moving residents, with sticks, zimmer frames and an occasional wheelchair.

8.30: Breakfast. Everyone is seated. The senior staff are behind the hatch serving the food; the assistants take it to the residents. Cereal or grapefruit, bread or toast, poached egg and baked beans. The residents are sitting four to a table; cutlery and china are standard, so are serviettes but each ring is marked with a name; there are cloths on the table. There is a teapot on each table and the group has usually decided who is going to pour. The meal is fairly quiet. Second helpings are taken round for those who want them. The clatter of dishes being washed up is heard. Some residents get up to go; others finish off their meal, talk, or wait for tablets which are taken round at the end of the meal. Some people have ordered a daily paper and these are handed round.

9.00: The residents make their way to the sitting rooms, some with staff assistance. One or two help others by collecting sticks or walking frames. A blind woman is seen to her room by a resident. Two or three residents go into the kitchen to finish the last of the drying-up. Most of the residents go to their particular places in the sitting areas. One or two in each room read the paper; some are already dozing; others will knit, sew, or chat.

10.30: The drinks trolley is taken round. Most residents stick to their regular drinks, milky coffee, coffee cooled with cold water, or squash. A lot of chatter between the assistant and the residents, about last night's TV programme, children at home, relatives' visits. One or two residents have been in their bedrooms, coming out when they hear the drinks come round.

Meanwhile some residents are being bathed – by two assistants if they are very heavy or frail, otherwise by one.

Letters are brought round by the secretary. One resident gets up to lay the tables for lunch; someone else has walked down to the town to place his daily bet. A woman calls in to see her father before she collects her children from school.

11.00: Bathing continues. Residents see a senior staff member as she goes to each sitting area in turn – 'What do you think about those tablets I have been given?'; 'How are you getting on with the plans for the coffee morning?'; 'Do you know if I am going out for the day on Sunday?' – she is asked.

Two people go to the nearby pub for a drink.

12.00: A start is made towards getting some residents ready for lunch. They are taken to the toilet or helped along to the dining hall. The more fit leave it until later to make a move.

12.30: Nearly everyone is sitting at the tables. Two are missing – one man is always late, but an assistant goes to look for the other person. It is a noisier meal than breakfast. Meals are served up at the hatch and carried round. A few people need their food cut up; someone doesn't like what she has got. A man gets up to go to the toilet. The second course is served. A similar pattern to breakfast – some wait for tablets, others leave, one or two dry the glasses.

1.00: Many have settled back in their armchairs. Several have gone to their bedrooms to lie down. The TV is on in one sitting room.

2.00: The afternoon is more leisurely than the morning. Cleaners have finished their work. Some people are bathed; others doze or listen to the radio. There are more visitors and more residents go out – to clubs or for a walk. Two people read books, several knit.

2.30: Tea is brought round on a trolley. The TV is put on in the men's sitting room for the racing.

5.00: High tea. The pattern is similar to other meals. There is a cooked main course followed by cakes and bread and butter.

6.15: Eight residents have met in the dining hall to play bingo. One of them calls the numbers. Later, a staff member takes over for a short time; the residents are glad when a visitor offers to call the numbers. Around the rest of the home the televisions are all on. There are more visitors. One or two people are bathed before bed.

7.15: An evening drinks trolley is taken round with a selection of hot milk drinks, squash and biscuits. Those who need help in getting to bed are taken to their rooms by the care assistants. Several others choose to go to bed soon after 8.00.

9.00: Most residents are in bed. Four of those who are still up gather in a sitting room near the office to chat and watch TV. Some men have stayed in their own sitting room upstairs. One man has been across to the pub.

10.00: Those who are downstairs have a cup of tea with staff. One by one they go to bed.

11.00: All residents are in their rooms. Some have had sleeping tablets. One or two may need to call staff during the night for help to get to the toilet.

CONTROL OF LIFE-STYLE

The key questions which are examined in this section are: 'How far is a resident able to decide how she will live?'; 'what factors exert influence on her life-style?'. The items selected as indicators (see above, pp. 32–3) are used as headings for this discussion.

(1) Money
All residents were expected to hand over their pension books to the secretary. She made arrangements to cash their weekly pension, would deduct the payment due to the local authority and distributed the remainder every Friday to residents in the sitting rooms. This was

termed 'pocket money'. Residents might keep all or part of this money, together with any other they might have. If they wished they could deposit money in the office for safe keeping. There was a notice in the wardrobe in each room stating that the local authority would take no responsibility for money missing from rooms.

Not all residents meekly submitted.

I was in the office when a hunchbacked, determined woman came in as a resident. The secretary asked her for her pension book so that she could change the designated post office, and also so that the matron would be granted authorisation to cash the pension. The resident would not hear of it. 'I won't sign anything; I'm going home soon' she said. 'She knows her own mind too well. You can't pull the wool over her eyes' said a senior staff member.

Another resident had to pay more than the minimum because of her assets. She did not like being at the home and found herself persuaded to stay there. Her anxiety about what was happening to her made her determined and she refused to pay anything except through her solicitor. Her solicitor was informed and he paid the bill. Later it transpired she had had enough money in her handbag to pay the bill. She had not been asked to give up her handbag, though staff suspected she might have had the money.

At any one period there were about three residents who were given no money because they were regarded as too confused and the money would then be placed in an account for them. If they were thought to need items such as toiletries or clothing it would be spent for them. It was assumed that residents did not understand what was going on. However, one resident commented: 'They used to keep my money in the office and buy me clothes, stockings and that', so she had been aware that her money was spent for her.

Some residents appeared to give most of the sum they had left (about £3) to their relatives. Staff would feel considerable anger towards such relatives, especially when they were thought to visit only to get the money. One man had a daughter who handled all his money and gave him what she considered he needed. He was left with very little. One day he told me how he had asked her for another pair of shoes. 'You've got a pair of shoes in your room', she replied, 'you don't need another.' 'I do really though', he added to me, 'because I keep doing wee on my shoes.' A woman was unable to pay to go out on outings or for a drink because she was left with so little.

On the other hand, residents who had few relatives and spent little might save a lot of money. One man had to be taken to hospital from the home. When he was about to go he handed over £516 which he had saved under his mattress. Had staff known about it, they would have banked it and this would have increased his capital to the point where he would have had to pay a larger contribution. The resident was as well aware of this as the staff. There were other occasions when staff found themselves with information about additional finances that residents had not declared. Staff felt torn between loyalty to the resident and to the local authority.

(2) *Cleaning*

Domestic workers were employed to clean the home. Expenditure cuts had meant these staff were employed for fewer hours so areas like the dining hall were polished less often. The significant factor here is that the bedrooms were cleaned each morning by domestic staff and residents were expected to keep out of their rooms until they were cleaned.

Care assistants made the beds. A few residents made their own, though some thought this was not allowed. No resident did any washing or ironing, though a few relatives did take clothes away to wash at home.

Several points emerged through considering this area. The domestic staff might grumble about rooms which they considered too untidy. Mrs Draxton moved into a single room. 'It was the first morning I was in my new room. I hadn't had time to get straight. My arm ached appalling. She [a domestic] came in – "I'm not having this room like this" she said. So this morning I got up and tried to get it tidy. "That's better, my dear" she said to me.' Another time Mrs Draxton was in trouble for leaving some clothes out on her bed and not putting them away in drawers.

There was no consultation with residents about how often they liked the room cleaned or how they liked it done. There seemed no encouragement to residents to consider doing it for themselves, in fact no joint planning about what was needed. This is significant in view of the fact that a survey of isolated elderly by Tunstall (1966) showed that cleaning was second only to cooking as the task carried out by most people at least once per week.

(3) *Clothing*

Residents had separate wardrobes and chests of drawers. Some clothes would be kept in these, some centrally in the linen room. Certain residents had more clothes kept centrally, but it was not possible to be certain whether these were the more confused residents (the stated reason) or the more passive ones. It is easier to keep clothes centrally than to distribute them around.

While the stated policy was that residents could change clothes whenever they wanted, some residents were said to abuse this. 'Could I have my red and black dress? I don't know where it is, it has been taken away' said Mrs Hughes. 'Yes, some of the summer ones were put away' was the reply from the care assistant, 'I'll see and come back if I can.' To me she added: 'I shan't do anything. We took her clothes away a few weeks ago because she kept changing them and putting them to the wash.' The effect of this type of deception could only be to disorient further someone who was already thought to be confused.

The general pattern was that residents could wear what they wanted and keep control of it. There were difficulties about sorting clothes – one man regularly confided that he was wearing someone else's pants – but while this was sometimes correct and partly accounted for by poor marking of clothes, there were times when he was mistaken. The standard of washing and ironing was high, though staff accepted there were occasional mistakes in sorting clothes.

Residents dressed differently and mostly chose what they wanted to wear. The control of staff was shown by their ability to control the quality of the service. While nearly all residents smelt fresh, Mr Gasden's clothes were not washed frequently enough and regularly he smelt of urine.

Two other incidents stand out. The first was a comment from a relative that her father had found it difficult to get used to life in the home 'because even on his own he used to like pottering around. He liked it a bit scruffy – in the home it was too clean, but *he eventually got used to a collar and tie,* etc.' This shows the way expectations become introduced. I had not picked up any mention that men had to wear ties; presumably this expectation was passed on to new residents and all the men ended up wearing ties. In the second incident two care assistants decided to snip a bit of lace off someone's nightdress ('she'll never notice') because they wanted it for a lavender bag to sell at a coffee morning to raise funds for the residents: an example of priorities getting so mixed up that an act of mild delinquency takes place.

(4) *Daily programme*

Residents were free to plan a large part of their day. However, this simple statement masks some of the more subtle influences. Residents were not allowed to stay in bed. There was anxiety amongst staff that once one person did that, everyone would want to. A senior staff member said: 'The doctor says Mrs Black needs to rest more. We'll put her to bed in the afternoons, perhaps that will help. Her niece was here and said "Couldn't she stay in bed, she'd be in bed at home". It is difficult to know when it's best to let them lie, sometimes it's not in their best interests. But she is 92 and I think she'd probably have got over it more quickly if she'd stayed in bed.'

Miss Johns, usually very compliant, said 'Sometimes I wish I could stay in bed longer', and others felt like her. Mrs Sidney was grateful that staff had persuaded her to get up when she felt depressed. 'You get so used to the routine. You are better for getting up. I don't mind getting up now' she said. Mrs Pinker, who was blind, was one of several who got up before being called.

> I'm happy about getting up; I woke about three-thirty a.m. yesterday and didn't sleep again. Got out and cleaned my teeth, tidied my drawer, back into bed and do some knitting. It passes the time – well I shouldn't wish the time away, mustn't say 'Oh I wish the day was over', it's wrong to wish that. I ought to like the day though, if I'm well and happy. If I was in pain or desperate I might feel different.
>
> I would get up at the time we do anyway. I start getting dressed and washed. Get up about seven-twenty and I'm ready by eight o'clock, it could be before that.

She went on to describe the rest of her day.

> Miss Johns comes and picks me up. I listen to the radio. Always have something at breakfast – the only trouble is that the toast isn't crisp, all steamy, doughy. Love to get to the dining hall and hear all the conversations.
>
> Then I go to the sitting room. Mostly knitting or talking, someone might read the paper to me. I like to hear people talking but I'm not used to talking to other people, not a conversationalist.
>
> You get a lot of fun from listening. You shut your eyes and listen, you'd be surprised what you hear. I knit on and off all day.
>
> Come in my room from dinner-time till half-past three, listen to my book, snooze, listen to the radio. The doctor says 'You should lay on your bed, it's advisable to rest'. I go back to the sitting room and knit, more knitting.
>
> Come to bed about eight o'clock. Some of the TV is confusing. I miss a lot. I like coming in to my room at night, being quiet, I don't get bored.

Mrs Pinker loved going to meals to hear all the bustle. When they were in the home, residents were usually expected to go in to meals. This served as a check on people's whereabouts and their eating habits.

Mrs Knight was well aware of staff expectations: 'I feel ill when I get up. Don't know how I get down to meals. They like you to go down if you can.'

Miss Manfield didn't mind getting up, but added: 'I get short of breath. Sometimes I don't care if I go to breakfast – I feel faint sometimes. Do you have to go to breakfast?'

There was some uncertainty about use of bedrooms. The problem was that domestics had to get in to clean rooms. Interpretations of what this meant varied. Senior staff members said that residents should be out while their rooms were cleaned; the norm appeared to be 'do not use bedrooms until 12 noon', while some residents genuinely thought they were not meant to go in their rooms at any time of the day.

Care assistants or domestic staff, anxious to get on with their work, might tell residents they were not meant to be in their rooms. Interestingly it was accepted that two residents did spend all day in their rooms. They were regarded as eccentric or stubborn and the cleaning went on round them. This is an illustration of the way in which stubbornness can lead to an individual modification of norms. It shows the importance for the elderly of asserting mastery – and that it is necessary to find socially acceptable ways of this happening.

With some other provisos, residents were free to plan their day. Visitors could come and go without making appointments; residents were free to go shopping, wander round the grounds or the town. Inevitably for many the constraints were to do with their own limited ability – there were variations from the fully mobile, to those walking short distances with zimmer frames, to people who needed staff assistance for any movement. Even given these increased dependencies, some chose to go out to clubs (when transport was arranged) while others did not.

Miss Carpenter liked to keep active and, though she needed a stick, was more active than most residents. She was glad of transport to take her to Red Cross meetings.

I look forward to the Sunday service, Gospel meetings, holidays and Red Cross. I like doing things for people, help Miss X down in the lift, wash up. I have tablets to take when I wake at about five in the morning. Get myself dressed – hope I always shall. I sit down in the lounge after breakfast – talk – sometimes go in and see Mrs Y. After lunch I read in my bedroom from about three-fifteen to four-fifteen. Sometimes there are entertainments or I watch TV. Two of the others decide what goes on.

It has already been mentioned that fit residents could go to bed when they wished. Those needing staff help had to be got ready earlier, and indeed got up in the morning earlier.

Mr Peat described his evening. 'After tea we watch TV – we all like the same sorts of things – go to bed about ten or ten-thirty.'

Mrs Smith similarly watched TV and then went to bed about eight-thirty. 'I don't want to stay up any longer and then I read in bed.'

Several residents described parts of the day that seemed boring. Some, like Mrs Knight, found physical handicap limited what they could do.

I don't like getting up because I can't stand long. Don't eat much breakfast. I make my bed myself. They know if I leave it that I can't manage it. I sit in the bedroom after breakfast – quiet till ten-thirty – I can't sew or knit. I read books in the morning. I don't talk a lot, like being quiet. I don't look forward to meals much. The doctor just says 'That's your old stomach complaint'. After lunch I have to sit quiet till half-past three, have to rest my legs which swell.

In spite of handicap she said that she didn't get bored.

Mrs Tanner clearly missed the activity of family life. She seemed happiest when there were things to do.

I used to get up at seven-thirty – the whole family did – granddaughter used to say 'Not coming down early again!'. I wouldn't get up quite so early now if I could choose; I just take a few minutes to get dressed and then I go straight down to breakfast. I strip my bed before breakfast and then make it, I don't like anyone else making my bed; it takes about fifteen minutes. I'm out of the room by nine-thirty. I read, but can't read all the time. Read the paper – then it's coffee. 'What, eleven o'clock already?' I think. The morning doesn't seem long.

Afternoons seem endless. Worse than the morning. Go out when it's nicer. Sometimes when I go out with my grand-daughter I walk home – up to the railway line – or go to the shops with her. Have visitors quite frequently, once or twice a week. In the evenings they have TV, silly programmes. I don't like westerns. I go to bed at nine o'clock. I used to stay up and watch the programmes but I'd be the only one. I like watching *Mastermind*, I like things like that that have some reality. Don't talk much, they don't like it. They're a dumb league in the afternoon. Don't play bingo because I can't see to play.

Staff were uncertain as to how far residents should be left when sitting passively. There were occasional attempts to interest them – one staff member tried to interest a resident in some magazines. Another would turn on the TV for residents – on one occasion when she left a resident said: 'Good, now we can turn it off; she always puts it on, though we don't want it.' Sometimes staff members tried to persuade residents to go out for a drink or do a puzzle. Mr Peters muttered to me that he didn't like doing puzzles but, perversely, seemed to get pleasure from having completed one.

Staff were also concerned to keep residents mobile. Residents had different opinions about how appropriate this was. Mrs Pinker described a very old resident, Mrs White, who was being made to walk. Someone who sat at her table thought it hard to keep pressing her. Mrs Pinker said: 'I think if you give up you'd give up for ever. If I thought I wouldn't do any knitting I could sit and mope.'

The tensions were focused most clearly when there were 'events' on. Although starting from a belief that residents were free to decide, pressures were often exerted on residents to attend, both for the sake of the 'performer' as well as from a belief that it would be good for the resident.

Mrs Quigley, Mrs Sidney and Miss Carpenter discussed the pending visit of someone who was coming to show them how to make Christmas decorations. Mrs Quigley: 'I think I'll go up to my room now. I don't want to go to that group this week.' Miss Carpenter: 'I don't want to go. I can't do anything with my hands.' Mrs Sidney: 'I shan't go either.' Before Mrs Quigley had left a senior staff member came in. 'Are you coming, Mrs Quigley?' 'Oh, all right then.' Miss Carpenter added: 'Well, I could just sit and watch.' Mrs Sidney chimed in 'I may have visitors', and she was very glad later to have a visitor and consequently a legitimate excuse.

It seemed at times that the church services in the home were boosted by the presence of the confused and the passive who would go along when directed.

(5) Bathing

Residents were bathed once a week. A record was kept of the date and comments were added about soreness or need for a chiropodist.

Most residents had got used to being bathed by other people, either relatives or district nurses, before coming into the home. The few who were embarrassed at the experience soon got used to it, helped by the staff attitude. Mrs White said: 'I'm used to it now though it was embarrassing. I know the girls. It's lovely to have a nice drop of water. A good many people never knew what it was like to have a bath.'

Nearly everybody was grateful for the help. Mrs Roberts, a large woman, who was often bathed by two staff, found that 'they jabbered to each other about their husbands'. She much preferred being bathed by one person. One day when I helped bath somebody I found similarly that the care assistant and I were talking to each other and the resident was being ignored.

While residents were glad to be helped they were often resentful about the timing. In spite of listening for cues' – 'I wonder if it will be my turn soon. Mrs Smith has had another bath since I have' – residents were often taken by surprise and did not like suddenly having to go off for a bath.

Mrs Richardson: 'It's my turn for a bath soon. I just said to my friend that I didn't really want one, not today. Still you can't tell them that. I'll feel better after I've had it. I don't like it when they bath me at twelve. That's too much of a rush before lunch. I thought they might do that today. Still I must be thankful they didn't bath me then.'

Mrs Sidney felt that 'you can't be too long because someone else needs to be helped'.

Mrs Smith said about another occasion: 'I never have got annoyed, only once. That was the other day. They came and took me for a bath in the evening. I prefer to be advised when, I had some visitors coming. I wouldn't say "no" but it is annoying.' This was in marked contrast with situations where staff took note of residents' feelings about times of bathing or gave some advance warning. 'All right for a bath in half an hour, Mr Gasden?'

One day when Mrs Williams had a bad cold she didn't think she should have a bath. The senior staff member thought she should. 'I've got to go and have a bath. I don't want to, still I suppose I've got to, got to obey orders.'

There was a firmness to the policy about bathing. Holiday visitors were bathed even when they protested that they had had a bath just before coming in.

It is, of course, unusual for most people to bath during the day. A large part of the stress for the residents was that they had to undress and dress again, a procedure that was often tiring. This raises the question as to whether changes in staffing hours or of times when residents get up would alleviate this.

(6) *Food*

At breakfast and tea, teapots, bread and butter and jam were placed on the table. The remainder of the meal was served on to plates in the kitchen and the care assistants took the meals to residents. They had a good knowledge of likes and dislikes ('Mrs Sidney won't have any gravy') but residents were dependent on the memory and concern of staff. Some residents were prepared to ask for a meal to be changed – 'I don't really want any potato today' – but most accepted what they were given. Some would add: 'It's not quite what I wanted, but I'll have it.'

The quality of the food was excellent and there was usually a choice of main course. Residents commented on how much they enjoyed it. Mr Murphy said: 'I enjoy the meals – too much, though. It's good and well cooked. They can't cook it how you would like it, though. Everything is cooked soft. I was more used to food in bigger lumps, pork chops and things.' Inevitably it was different from what people were used to (there was more or less salt) and the difficulty of adjusting to this highlights the significance of food. Food seems the symbol of the intimacy of their past life and at least as significant to men as to women.

The fact of being waited on by staff is also important. Restaurants and hotels are the situations when we expect to be waited on, and there is a strange duality in this relationship. The customer has the power to select what he requires but also feels very dependent. 'Shall I ask for more milk?' 'Will the waiter be surly or pleasant?' 'We have waited here for hours.' 'Shh, dear, don't make a fuss.' Those comments reflect some of the uncertainty. In the old age home the power of the customer is reduced (he is not paying a bill in the same way), while that of the person serving seems greatly increased. The care assistant has knowledge of most of a resident's life and considerable power in other spheres of living. It is not so easy to assert yourself. Early in my research notes I described this as 'the powerlessness of the hotel guest'.

In fact there was little formal pressure on residents to eat particular foods. They could eat just vegetables or no vegetables at all. Yet there was a reluctance to leave residents with their choices. 'I should have a bit of meat' said a care assistant. At its extreme this could lead to feeding by staff.

Mr Page came in to lunch. He looked dishevelled and was not well. He had brought a bottle of beer in with him. He was deaf and often would not use a hearing aid, which made little difference. Staff poured out his beer for him; he turned down any food. The care assistant put his bib on him and tried to push the food in. 'You must have something, it's good for you.' Most of it dribbled down his chin. Later another care assistant tried: 'Matron says you have got to have this sweet.' He pushed it away: 'I'll have it for tea.' There was a discussion between staff and residents. 'He needs his food, he'll get weak without it . . . '

I was surprised on my first day at the large helpings of food eaten by residents and even more surprised to see residents consuming second helpings of the first course. Clearly I was wrong to have assumed that the old would eat less. There was another side, however. 'Matron likes to see you eat a lot' said Mrs Smith.

An example:

SENIOR STAFF MEMBER TO MRS ROBERTS: 'You'll have some more custard and apple. Here Mr Clough, give it to her.'
MRS ROBERTS: 'No, thank you.'
STAFF MEMBER: 'Yes she will, put it down.'
ME: 'Would you?'
MRS ROBERTS: 'Not really.'
STAFF MEMBER: 'Go on, put it there, she'll have it.'
Mrs Roberts had pushed her plate away, but said reluctantly: 'Well, I'll see what I can do.' Presumably it is very satisfying for staff to see residents enjoying their food.

Timing of attendance at meals is also a visible reminder of one's status. Mrs Williams disliked waiting before a meal. 'It's like schoolchildren; still you've got to put those things aside.' It was noticeable that the fittest came last to meals. Residents attached importance to getting to meals on time. Meals were served at set times: 8.30 a.m., 12.30 p.m. and 5.00 p.m. 'I'm afraid for my life of being late' said

Miss Brinton. 'I don't think I'd get any if I came late, though people are excused.' Other residents expressed similar anxieties.

There was an expectation that residents would come in to meals if they were in the home. Recognised illness was a legitimate excuse; the visit of a relative was grudgingly accepted. Otherwise people were persuaded to come in and 'just sit', or 'just eat a little'. Meal-times provided a check on the whereabouts of residents. Provided they had stated they were going out, residents were perfectly free to miss meals.

Another aspect of the method of serving was that there were frequent shouts across the dining hall – 'Gravy, Mrs Sidney?' – especially to certain residents who were more assertive. By contrast one care assistant would go round the table in advance asking what was wanted. 'I do like to be asked, not just have a meal put down' said Mrs Tanner.

Having served the meal, staff appeared to stand round like vultures waiting to pounce on empty plates. Residents must have felt the rush and few stayed chatting at the end of the meal.

It is easy to forget that the freedom to manage life-style is not constrained only by staff. It is constrained also by other residents. I had been prepared for worse table manners than I saw. In spite of the fact that behaviour was nearer normal than I had expected, bad table manners were mentioned by residents most often as the most annoying behaviour of others. There were comments like 'I shouldn't want to eat at some tables'; 'table habits are annoying'; 'Mr Page coughs at the table'; 'I have to tell them not to do some things'. The extreme situation was rare – a member of staff described a meal when one man said he couldn't sit and watch another eat, while a different man was spitting away.

Residents would exert direct control on behaviour. Mrs Richardson described such an event: 'I went to pour a second cup of tea one evening and he said "You are in a temper". I said "Indeed not, don't say that about me". No one must touch the teapot when he is about. He is ninety-two years of age and he shakes some tea in the saucer sometimes.'

But meals provided positive stimulation also: 'I love to get down to the dining hall and hear all the conversations'; 'there's something nice about going down to meals – you all meet together again and the attendants are ready to serve us'; 'I enjoy meals, hearing what everybody is saying', said three residents.

(7) *Medical services*
Residents were able to choose their own doctor. This was important to them. The procedure was that if they felt ill or wished to see the doctor they would ask the staff to make arrangements. This gave staff some power of interpretation as to whether a doctor was needed or not. Mrs Williams used to get her son to take her out to the doctor's

surgery because 'I get the feeling they [the staff] think I'm making a fuss'. She was the only person who went out to see a doctor.

There were other examples of the constraints imposed by this system. In the first a senior staff member decided that it was not necessary to call the doctor for two residents who had asked to see him; in the second, about a different resident, Mrs Sidney stated: 'They should have called the doctor days ago.'

The doctor usually saw the patient in a bedroom, though there were a few occasions when doctors carried out a consultation in a sitting room with other residents around.

The regulations of the local authority stated that all medicines and drugs were to be kept by the staff unless a doctor specified otherwise. In fact all drugs were held centrally and distributed at the end of meals, though a few residents did buy occasional cough sweets or Aspro. This meant that residents did not keep their own drugs.

Medicines themselves exerted a considerable control over life-style, both beneficial and harmful. The beneficial aspect was in alleviating pain and controlling chronic conditions; the harmful side was that, in spite of attempts by staff and occasionally by doctors, there was a general agreement that residents ended up with too many tablets, and this might lead to the residents' confusion. Some staff felt that sometimes antibiotics were used inappropriately and led to a slower, more painful death. Residents were often uncertain about the value of their medication. Mr Jepson complained about the tablets he was taking: 'It's not worth having them if they make you feel so rotten. I'd rather die.'

(8) Furniture and decorating

Residents were allowed to take in small possessions, including a chair and commode. There was little room for anything else and no opportunity to store the furniture of the home. The position of the bed, central with access on both sides, made for convenience in making beds. Many people in bed-sitters would have a bed against the walls where it functions more like a couch. Most rooms had only a few bits and pieces around. There was little that made a permanent feeling of possession, for example, pictures hung on the walls. People were allowed to carpet their bedrooms but the carpet had to stay when a resident left or died. No resident had had her room painted or decorated to suit her own taste.

The personality of the resident would influence the amount of control that was exerted on her to keep the room tidy. Some rooms on the ground floor were passed by all visitors coming into the home and there seemed greater pressure for these to be kept tidy. A determined resident would be able to have a lot of clutter around.

In each room there was a small drawer with a lock in the bedside cupboard. The keys of some of these had been lost, leaving some people with nowhere to lock anything up. The request of one man to fit a lock to his wardrobe was turned down by a senior staff member.

It has already been noted that residents were not supposed to be in their rooms at certain times.

These indicators of resident control proved useful. While their links to the typology of homes will not be made until Chapter 11, the indicators allow comparison with other styles of living.

NEEDS AND RESOURCES

Let us take the case of a resident who was living in her own house prior to admission. There would be limitations also on her ability to control her life-style in areas discussed above (bathing, cleaning, etc.). It would be necessary to take account of her resources – health, money, housing, access to support. Thus she might be too handicapped to cook a meal and consequently dependent on someone cooking for her. Similar examples could be multiplied in relation to any of the other headings.

The significant difference between the two life-styles is that in the old age home resources are made available to meet needs. However, the more resources a resident needs, the more she is likely to lose control of the manner in which those resources should be provided. Gubrium suggests that satisfaction is dependent on a balance between activity resources and activity norms. Therefore if an individual has the resources available to match the expectations of the immediate society in which she lives (including her own expectations) then she can be said to be coping.

Transfer to a residential home profoundly alters the balance between resources and norms. The resources side of the equation receives a sudden boost. The individual is freed from some of the anxieties of daily living – paying bills, keeping the house warm – and receives help with meeting personal needs – bathing and feeding. Consequently she has more time, and may be in better health, to do other things. But at the same time the other side of the equation, the norms or the expectations of those around her, also alter. The past balance goes haywire and a new harmony needs to be established. It is crucial to realise that there are positives for the resident through the provision of additional resources; yet, grateful as residents may be for those resources, in situations where they have minimal control over the way the resource is provided they are often uneasy.

PUBLIC AND PRIVATE

It is difficult to capture the key elements of life in an old age institution. A comparison with other styles of living is helpful. The normal pattern of living in society is to live on one's own or in a small group. This group is more or less secluded from the rest of the community and there are clear boundaries between the group and the outside. Inside the individuals eat, sleep, relax. They emerge when they wish to meet other people, go to work, play, or for any other reason; similarly they may invite others into their base. One of the essential changes for an individual in an old age institution is that the privacy of the base is lost.

This is of fundamental importance. Between the inside and outside of one's own home is a clear boundary, however often it may be crossed. Is the resident to see the base as her own room, or the whole institution? The first is too small and, in this establishment at least, not a private living base; the latter is too large, too public and too diffuse. Mrs Pinker had lived in the country before admission. She had lived in a row of houses and would stop and speak to people. She never had anyone into her house and never went into another house. In a way she thought she lost contact with the outside world. But within her house she had been very happy with her husband and children, and her whole life had centred on them and her garden. It was hard for her to transfer to a situation where there was no clear inside base and outside world.

It may be possible to make the individual's room in the old age home approximate more closely to this idea of a base. At The Pines there were severe limitations. Staff would enter rooms without knocking except for the very first call of the day. They would go into cupboards to take out or put clothes away; the cleaners would similarly go in when they needed to. When Mr Fothergill thought he was losing things he asked whether he might have a lock on his wardrobe. A senior staff member thought this highly inappropriate. 'What would the staff think if the residents began to lock things up? They would imagine they were not trusted.' Perhaps to begin to serve the function of a base residents would need to be able to lock the doors of the rooms.

An additional factor in the different living-styles concerns use of bedrooms. It has already been noted that residents were expected not to use the rooms until the cleaners had finished. However, some residents believed they were not supposed to use the rooms at any time. Others clearly felt that staff wanted them to come out and sit in the sitting rooms. Two residents did use their rooms as their regular base (they achieved this by ignoring the cajoling and persuading of staff). The rest used the sitting room as the normal living place and their rooms more as a bolt-hole, when they wanted a sleep or to receive visitors.

The result was that most people lived their lives in public in a way

they never had before (a few had experienced far more public living –
in the army or other institutions). They would sit and read, or knit,
or chat, or doze alongside other people. These experiences are shared
usually only in one's intimate living group. Here they were shared with
people they had not selected as friends.

Lipman (1968) comes to similar conclusions:

> Before field studies started it was assumed that the residents' bed-
> rooms would be venues for receiving fellow residents, that the
> designation 'bed-sitting room' given by the Ministry of Health ...
> indicated that some social life would take place in the bedrooms
> ... social life in the homes took place almost exclusively in the
> sitting rooms, and, to a lesser extent, in the dining rooms. The
> sitting rooms were the centres, the cockpits of social life in the Homes.

It is in this context, he argues, that it is necessary to consider the
way individuals develop 'rights' to particular chairs and places. 'It
seems that a person regularly occupying a chair exercises his authority
to exist as a social entity – his identity – in a physical location ... In
other words, the chair becomes a symbol of the occupant's social
existence ... '

In The Pines, as in many other old age institutions, residents did
exercise rights to particular chairs. Clearly this was linked to the fact
that the sitting room was the centre of social life but it is also linked
to the uncertainty about one's base.

Two further points make this uncertainty even more significant. The
first is the style of sitting rooms in the home. Since they were open-
plan with one side open to the corridor, living in the sitting room
meant that one was also living in a corridor. Thus people passing by
had to be greeted and acknowledged and might drop in for a chat.
Secondly, since the tasks of daily living were being carried out by the
staff, the resident had more time than ever before for 'non-work' activity.
Consequently, instead of living in comparative seclusion and emerging to
meet friends or to shop, the pattern for residents was to live in a semi-
public group and to retreat when separateness was wanted.

Therefore boundaries did not have the same significance. Nor were
residents protected by the boundary in the same way. Playing host to
friends means inviting them to cross into one's base, but at The Pines
friends would come in uninvited. The resident was no longer able to play
host, nor to refuse to see unwelcome visitors. So the very freedom of
visitors to drop in when they wished and without letting staff know,
a freedom that was positively welcomed by most residents, created
further changes in living-style. It would be difficult to find ways of
fulfilling the role of host or of protecting the resident.

At The Pines the visitor assumed most of the power that normally
belongs to the host. Many visitors chose to talk to their friend or

relative in the sitting room. Often there was no spare chair on which they might sit. The fact that they were standing heightened the passivity of the old person, and it was often the visitor who initiated conversation with others in the room. The role of the host in receiving, settling and providing for the visitor largely disappeared.

Occasional comments point to the fact that visitors, usually other people's, could be intrusive. Mrs Sidney commented that she would go somewhere else when this happened. Most visitors had a specific purpose, that of visiting a particular resident. There was little need for protection from these. On the other hand intrusions from staff, other residents, or interested people were not so easy to handle.

I was aware of this problem and did not find it easy to walk into a sitting area and begin conversation. Residents are a captive audience who have become used to receiving whoever wishes to walk in. I felt that it would be difficult for them to find a way of showing me that they did not wish for my company. For example, I might go into a sitting area, chat to one person and find other people putting down the books they had been reading. Would they rather have been left in quiet? These feelings are echoed by a resident, Mrs Richardson, who said in interview: 'I don't go and visit in other lounges. I don't know whether they appreciate me coming or not. So I stopped visiting, though I have visited about three times.' And it was echoed also by a health visitor, replying to a question about visiting residents. 'It's a chore, embarrassed about whether or not to chat to other residents' she wrote.

My solution was to make a point of asking whether it was all right to sit down and then weigh up whether I was in the way or not. I found that I went more to the four sitting areas which were on corridors (1, 2, 3 and 5, Figures 6.1 and 2) because it was easier to walk past if people were sleeping or busy. The day before I left the home I heard from a senior staff member that the residents in sitting area 4 had been complaining that they never saw me, and had been aware that I went more often to other areas. I explained the dilemma to them and that others had more often invited me to stop and talk. However, the issue of being available without imposing and without reinforcing the dependent role of the resident is real.

In addition to uncertainty about boundaries, another aspect of public living is sharing in one's life. Goffman (1961) gives examples of this from a range of establishments, and I recorded several forms at The Pines.

Residents might feel that other people were listening to all that was going on. Mrs Loosely was talking to me in the sitting room. Several times she said 'You see, there's no privacy' and followed that later with 'They're talking about us'. Yet she did not want to move into the bedroom for the pattern of using the sitting room was so firmly established. I did not know whether the two people talking at the far end of the room had been talking about us or not. Mrs Loosely's hearing was very good and she may well have been right. A few days later as I talked with her she asked: 'Are they talking about us? That's the trouble here – all your business is known.'

There was no doubt that all your business was known. Most of it was transacted in front of other people, and the rest they would hear commented upon. Miss Carrow had had a fall and broken her arm. She was feeling bemused one day when she had a letter from a relative which recounted an incident on holiday. Miss Carrow got this incident out of its real perspective and worried about it for much of the day. Miss Carpenter and Mrs Sidney watched her from the other end of the room. 'There you are you see. She's picked up that letter again. Watch her, look. There, holding it again.'

While there may be much that people are willing to share, there are episodes that they want to keep private. Goffman points out how the normal pattern is to move out from home, to work, to yet another base for leisure or club activities. With each move parts can be left behind that one does not want to share in the new situation. Residential living exposes the individual in all areas. In particular the indignities suffered by residents are witnessed by others. 'You should have gone before lunch' said a staff member to a resident as he went to the lavatory during the meal. Everybody around him would see him slightly demeaned.

Indignities, of course, were by no means always staff-induced. Residents' own silly or stubborn behaviour would also be made public. Even more worrying for them was when they began to lose control over their bodies. Mr Gasden went through a spell when he was wet every evening. Fortunately a staff member realised that he was embarrassed about moving while other people were up because they would see his wet trousers – and she let him stay up until after the others had gone to bed. Mr Jepson was not so lucky. He was wet in the middle of lunch, was told to go off and change, and came back after the others had finished their meal and sat and cried. On another day Mr Fothergill had soiled his trousers. He offered one of the care assistants 50 pence if she would keep quiet about it.

So it is rather more than others knowing one's interests. They know intimate details about one's physical and emotional state. It may be hard to remember that such information ought to be used with utmost discretion. Staff at The Pines sometimes seemed to have forgotten this. They would talk to staff about residents in the hearing of other residents. At its most extreme this would mean comments such as 'He's an evil old person' and, worse, 'Mr McNab has just made a mess upstairs and trodden in it – it's like looking after pigs'. A final example results more from thoughtlessness – a domestic assistant knew that Mr Peters had once cut his wrists in a suicide attempt. Seeing his room-mate's razor around, she said, with residents listening: 'Don't leave Mr Peat's razor lying around; you never know what Mr Peters might do.'

Indiscretion may result from lack of awareness or frustration or tiredness. Staff, on becoming exasperated with a resident, sometimes told other residents about it. A general comment in front of a group of residents was made by a staff member about a resident who was not going to be given a drink because on an earlier occasion she had not finished her drink: 'She's naughty with it, she doesn't half play up.' A few moments later, on meeting another resident, the staff member said to her 'That Mrs Hughes is playing up again'.

Such indiscretion may result from lack of awareness of the effect of one's actions or an inability to sense what others are feeling. In other words, it may not be deliberate harshness or insensitivity. The implication for staff training is that ways must be found to help staff realise the significance of seemingly small events to a resident.

Finally, public living means it is difficult to take life at one's own pace. It is not easy to make a quiet start to the day when bombarded with hearty greetings.

Effects of public living

Another aspect of public living is that events are conspicuous to all. Mrs Smith had a doctor to visit her one day. The doctor had to walk past another sitting room before reaching her room. In the sitting room that he passed a conversation began amongst residents about how often their own doctor visited. There was no doubt that being visited by a doctor conferred some status and therefore when Mrs Richardson said 'My doctor visits once a month whether I ask for him or not' others became uneasy.

Having visitors seemed to confer status also. Thus Mrs Williams would spend time talking about going out to friends and about the people who were calling to see her that day and the next day. There was enough of a pattern about this and similar events to suggest that she and others needed to build up a picture of life outside the home to impress residents.

The more public the style of living, the more the picture of self-worth seems dependent on ways of maintaining status. There were other ways in which this occurred. A common one was to tell off other residents: 'Don't interrupt, Miss Hacket' said Mrs Sidney in the sitting room. When the drinks trolley was taken round a resident would sometimes ask another 'What will you have?' to be met by the rejoinder 'I shall wait till I'm asked'.

The bad table manners of others have already been mentioned. While it was apparent why some habits were objectionable, there were other situations where the speaker seemed anxious to establish her own position, rather than to comment on the other person. Mr Fothergill described how some people ate from their knives instead of their forks and made it clear that he was used to being with a different sort of person. There were other occasions when he felt the need to establish himself as a worthwhile person. Then he talked about the standing of people he had known in a local town and the respect in which he had been held.

Some residents similarly made comments about others to establish their own position. Miss Carpenter at the table said to Miss Black, who was anxious as to whether her meal had been forgotten, 'Just wait, be patient'. And later, 'Just wait dear, she'll come to you. Oh, some people!' This seemed primarily a way of indicating her own patience and good behaviour.

Thus a part of the explanation for residents' behaviour is the maintenance of self-worth. Another aspect concerns expectations. Tobin and Lieberman's (1976) idea of 'anticipatory institutionalisation' has already been mentioned. They suggest that *in anticipation* of a move to a residential home old people change their picture of themselves, their roles and their capacities. This process is continued within the home when people have to 'manage' the state of being a resident. So people do not just exist and behave without considering their surroundings. They present themselves in ways that they think appropriate, in the same way as people do in any other situation. This is why I tried to find out what picture was held of a good resident.

I asked residents for their own interpretation and the view they thought was held by the staff. They failed to make this distinction and only half of the respondents answered this question. Most people thought 'tolerance' important and most of those characteristics mentioned were passive – 'falling in with everything', 'agreeing with most things', 'contented'. A few answers picked on attributes that were more active – 'being happy', 'being lively', 'being sociable' and 'trying to help'. One person commented that staff expect a resident to join in with things, and 'to be taken out of yourself'.

By contrast the 'bad' resident was described as 'ungrateful', 'miserable', 'moaner', 'disagreeable'; other points mentioned were people who 'chatted about others', and those 'who were inclined to be quarrelsome'. Some of the uncertainties as to the purpose of residential living are contained here. Should residents be expected to be sociable, to join in and even to show gratitude? In spite of uncertainty residents have developed an idea of how they ought to behave, and have started this construction before admission.

THE GAINS AND LOSSES OF RESIDENTIAL LIVING

So far in this chapter there has been an attempt to illustrate the style of living in an old age home by considering procedures (for example, in getting people up or providing meals) and by considering the public aspect of residential living. The constraints and the problems outlined are real and many of them are remediable. It is important at this stage to repeat an earlier statement that the constraints of residential living must not blind us to the constraints of other life-styles. Before admission many residents found their lives restricted and burdened. Entry to a residential home may be preferable to earlier living.

A brochure produced by the local authority (Somerset County Council, 1975) lists some of the pros and cons:

Obviously, when you are living with a large group of people – say 36 or 50 residents in all – it is difficult to provide a truly homely atmosphere. Nevertheless, every effort is made to encourage residents to create their own private living-space and their own individual way of life and staff are very aware of the importance of these needs. In our newer homes most of the residents have a room of their own – this helps.

WHAT DO I GAIN, WHAT DO I LOSE?

You gain by not having to worry about such things as: heating, lighting and cooking arrangements – repairs and replacements to property and furniture – how to get help quickly when you need it.

You have the ready-made companionship of the other residents and a large number of people from which to choose your friends. Skilled care is available at all times, night and day, and the building has been designed or adapted to meet the special needs of elderly people.

Inevitably, there are some disadvantages and there are some sacrifices to be made.

As in any community some loss of privacy is involved and a few restrictions are necessary. Almost certainly you will not be able to take with you all your personal possessions. The Head of the Home however helps people to decide what personal belongings can be accommodated. It is not usually possible for large items of furniture to be brought, but such things as pictures, photographs, ornaments, dressing table sets and even fireside chairs, desks and occasional tables can be and frequently are fitted in. More and more residents are arranging to have their rooms close carpeted and to have one or more of the walls of their room papered.

You will also need to adjust to a routine that the staff will make as flexible as possible, but may not be the one you would choose for yourself.

If you are sharing a room there is a need to consider other people in such things as playing the transistor radio and coming in late at night. Residents are, however, free to come and go as they please and are in fact encouraged to have a life outside of the Home. There are no curfews in our establishments. All the staff ask is that if you plan to be away for a meal or a night you should tell them, as otherwise they will worry about you and start searching for you.

It is also necessary that all drugs and medicines are handed to the Matron for safe-keeping. As certain drugs are dangerous if taken after alcohol, it is wise, in your own interest, to inform the Matron if you are accustomed to taking alcoholic drinks.

It is very important that NO SMOKING takes place in bedrooms as it is far too dangerous and places are set aside in the Home for smoking.

Our staff are aware of the snags and of the problems faced by the residents and they do try very hard to help and give a personal service.

Only you can judge if this kind of life is the best that is available to you. We believe that for a great many it is the best answer.

Most residents at The Pines thought they had made the right decision and twenty-two out of twenty-three respondents stressed that they would advise a friend to live in a residential home. There were three or four provisos to this – 'If there was nothing else to do' said one person, 'if you couldn't do the work' said another, while a third said 'if you had nobody to rely on'. The reasons for this nearly all fell into the areas covered by one of the paragraphs from the brochure. 'You gain by not having to worry about such things as: heating, lighting and cooking arrangements – repairs and replacements to property and furniture – how to get help quickly when you need it.'

Mrs Richardson expressed this clearly. 'The most important thing was feeling comfortable – nothing to worry about. I was able to rest, I'd done my duty. I was surprised at such a place.'

Residents were glad to have people to do things for them – washing, ironing, helping with getting to bed, bathing, dressing, doing errands. The other area that was mentioned by several people was that of having staff around. 'To have someone around', 'someone able to give you attention', 'somebody there when you're ill', 'bells' (to ring if assistance was needed) were some of the points mentioned.

When asked what they enjoyed most about living in a residential home most answers were to do with 'comfort', 'peacefulness', 'rest' and the provision of services. The kindness of staff was mentioned: 'nothing is too much trouble'.

A similar question was asked by Peace et al. (1979). They found that residents, when asked the one thing they liked best about living in the home, stated: a room of one's own (24 replies), material comforts (20), the care and attention (20), being looked after (20), the staff (11), the 'home from home' atmosphere (9), matron (5).

It is significant that activities were not mentioned in this list and at The Pines, where residents were not limited to one answer, only Miss Carpenter stressed activities as the most enjoyable factor. She said that she enjoyed the TV, entertainments, Christmas ('I enjoyed that very much indeed'), birthdays ('they all sing to you'). While others mentioned activities such as watching slide shows as enjoyable, nobody else stated activities were the best part of residential living. It would seem that such a life-style is regarded as freeing *from* burdens rather than freeing *to* do other things.

This is probably significant in relation to companionship and friendship. The fact has been mentioned that many residents stated the importance of having people around to help. This provides freedom *from* anxiety about what would happen if they fell and were alone, or were ill. Only Mrs Tanner mentioned company as one of the positives and she found a childhood friend in the home. Most stated that they did not have a special friend and this is similar to Townsend's (1962) findings.

These examples suggest how important it is to distinguish between social isolation and loneliness in old age. People who were unmarried and had led an isolated life tended not to complain about loneliness unless they had lost contact with a close friend. Those who had lost or been separated from someone they loved often felt lonely even when they had lived with other people. In fact the majority seemed to feel their loss more keenly, because there were fewer opportunities of losing themselves in household activities and relationships with other members of their families and friends.

People who are separated from past significant relationships (particularly spouse or children) do not expect to replace those by new deep relationships. However, companionship may help to make other losses bearable. In talking about friendship residents were clear that they had no special friends. One resident stated that she did not like to pick out one person for attention, another that she never had had special friends. However, the style of public living may lead people to question the attitudes of others towards them. For example, Mrs Knight said: 'None are close friends, they are acquaintances. It's hard to tell who your friends are. I hear quickly – and hear a lot of things I'm not meant to.' (She did add that she felt the same uncertainty outside.)

Mrs Draxton said that there was one person she thought she had made friends with but now she was not so sure. Living from a public base – the sitting area – means that others are seen over long periods, not just when one chooses and this fact, together with the jealousy that occurs when residents observe the activities of others, seems to discourage the forming of close relationships. Townsend (1962) found that 'fewer friendships were formed between persons sleeping in one room than between persons sleeping in single rooms'. Privacy may increase the likelihood of relationships being formed.

It is also important to note that only one person stated she was lonely 'quite often'. Most claimed they were never lonely and here there was frequent mention of other people: 'never lonely – there are always people around'; 'not at all lonely – so many people'; 'I'm lonely when I'm depressed, but there are people around'. The presence of other people reduced loneliness.

Two residents mentioned that the other residents were not the sort of people they would have chosen to live with, and it should be noted that residents had virtually no choice of where they sat in the dining hall or in sitting rooms. There were few situations where one might meet residents other than those from one's table or sitting area. Bingo was one of the few events where this happened.

The aspect of living with other residents that was disliked most was bad manners. However, some people who 'poked their noses in', were 'too religious', or 'too filthy in their talk' caused offence as well. Most stated they were not concerned about confused residents – 'you feel sorry for them' – though one or two incidents of wandering or finding a strange person in one's bed had been frightening. There was little problem about losing possessions, though one man recounted sharing a bedroom with a man who

didn't know what was his and someone else's. It can be very uncomfortable like that. You just make sure you don't lose too much. One chap I think had been a professional burglar! Still staff will get things back. He used to get up at three in the morning and I'd think, 'Now what's he up to ?'.

Inevitably some people found it difficult to live with others; on such occasions staff might move one of the residents. In the meantime the tension was considerable and Mrs Williams described how one resident had taken everything out of her hands. 'She was the same at the table in the beginning. "You don't want to do that. There's attendants to do that." One day I nearly ran away – it was all too much.'

One factor that surprised the residents was that there were few restrictions. They were pleased to have visitors when they wanted and the more active would go out for a walk or shopping without having to tell staff where they were going.

TASKS IN RESIDENTIAL LIVING

Townsend (1972) distinguishes three systems of occupation for inmates. 'Two are formally organised in institutions by the management. These are maintenance work of various kinds and occupational instruction or "therapy".' The third system is personal services among inmates.

(1) Maintenance work

This phrase is used to indicate work that is essential to the basic running of the establishment. Half-a-dozen residents would sometimes help with drying up, usually two after each meal. These residents would finish their meal and then dry up the few items that had not been finished. There were times when the request for help from staff was met grudgingly. A senior staff member asked Miss Carpenter to help dry up. 'Oh, my arthritis, I don't know' was the reply. Later Miss Carpenter said to two other residents: 'She asked me to dry up but I can't because of my legs.' Later still she was drying up. Usually residents were glad to help. It was a sign of their greater ability and it allowed them into a domain (the kitchen) that was exclusive to staff on most occasions; it allowed them also to meet residents from different sitting rooms and tables. Mrs Williams dried up and listened to the staff conversation. She smiled and said to me: 'I have lots of laughter just noticing what goes on.'

I was surprised that residents did nothing to clear the tables. In fact the reason probably was that staff cleared items away so promptly that there was little for the residents to do.

Miss Johns was the only resident who made a significant contribution to the running of the home. She laid up the tables for lunch and tea; often collected the cups after drinks had been taken round and washed them up. She was younger than most other residents, only 67, and had been transferred from the old workhouse. The care assistants were grateful for her help and gave her a special Christmas present.

Other help was only slight. Some residents made their beds, a few did some dusting. Mrs Richardson occasionally buttered some bread for tea. Mrs Quigley saw something was spilt in the sitting area and went to get a brush and dustpan – which was most unusual. Involvement in any tasks to do with running the establishment was slight. A few residents did a little. There is, of course, no clear picture as to the demands that ought to be made on residents. However, Tunstall (1966) showed that with his sample housework was the activity that provided the second most pleasure. Consequently there may be a link between the purposelessness felt by some residents and the minimal involvement (non-existent for most residents) in the running of the establishment. It is significant also that residents probably had more time available and less that they *needed* to do than at any other time in their adult lives.

(2) Occupational instruction

There were two occasions when someone came to teach the residents how to make Christmas decorations. These were the only examples of occupational instruction because the home had not got the services of an occupational therapist.

(3) *Personal services among inmates*

Initially I was struck by the passivity of residents and the little amount of help they gave to one another. In fact more thorough investigation showed a much larger system of helping than had been imagined. At meals some residents would collect the sticks and zimmer frames of others and place them out of the way. Miss Tippitt wiped the chairs and helped two residents who sat at her table. Mrs Quigley agreed to mend a dress for Mrs Sidney. She asked Miss Hacket to collect it from the bedroom since Miss Hacket shared with Mrs Sidney. Mrs Quigley then mended it. A staff member, incidentally, said: 'You needn't have bothered to do that. We'd have done it for her.' Some more able people were willing to get things for others. Mrs Pinker was blind and Mrs Smith would read the paper to her and help when she got stuck with her knitting. Mrs Richardson put a hot water bottle on the chair of a day visitor each day to warm it up for her. It was common for one resident to attract the attention of a staff member for another; similarly they would remind each other that it was time for tea, or time to come out of the bedroom to collect a drink. At night-time if they heard someone fall they might ring their alarm bell to attract the staff.

However, there was a clear understanding that residents should not help each other with moving about. Residents stated the reason was the staff fear that both helper and helped might fall, so making the situation worse. Mrs Williams was one of several who said how hard it was to see other people struggle and to do nothing. In fact she said one day that she had been helping the sick, 'though I know I'm not meant to'. On another occasion Mrs Quigley helped Mrs White stand up to go off to the toilet. She explained what she had done to a care assistant. 'I just helped her up. She has walked along to the toilet and she'll call you when she needs you.'

Townsend (1972) found that the infirm were less likely to help others and this was the case also at The Pines, though some of the more able performed no services for others.

PROVISION OF FACILITIES

Staff in a residential home have to decide how many facilities to provide on the premises. Cost may be one factor to consider but the more difficult one is whether residents should be encouraged to look outside the home for their needs.

At The Pines a small stock of goods was kept and taken round to residents about twice a week. The stock included sweets, cigarettes and toiletries. Mrs Quigley and Miss Carpenter started just before I left to take the trolley-load of goods round the home; until then it had been taken by a staff member. How well stocked should such a 'shop' be?

A hairdresser came regularly once or twice a week and residents were very grateful for the service, which boosted their self-image.

Posting letters was more difficult, since there was no postbox on the premises. Mrs Richardson would leave her letters prominently on the coffee table and wait for a staff member to ask 'Does this need posting?'. She would need to check up to ensure that the letter really had been posted. In fact a postbox would have made her less dependent on staff, for she could have posted the letters in an internal box herself and been more confident that they would not be forgotten, since it would have been emptied by the postman. So perhaps the difficult question should be tackled by the extent to which provision of facilities increases the independence of residents.

Mrs Roberts wished there was a phone in a place that was comfortable and private. Residents were dependent for incoming calls on staff passing on messages or staff calling them to the phone in the office to receive a call and were unable to phone anybody themselves unless in exceptional circumstances they asked to use the office phone. Staff were often willing to make arrangements for residents – they phoned for a taxi for Mrs Richardson – but residents remained unnecessarily dependent.

Indeed, an additional indicator of residential life, and one not used in this study, is *accessibility to the outside world*. This would document procedures for visitors (notices, arrangements, hours, privacy) and the residents' access to the outside (arrangements for posting and receiving letters, use of phone, spending time outside the home). This indicator might provide some clues to staff attitudes to residents. Accessibility to the world outside a residential establishment is significant in most institutions. Relatives and patients are concerned about times and conditions for hospital visiting. Anxiety about the posting of letters had been an important factor in the lead-up to riots at two boys' approved schools (HMSO, 1947, 1959). There were differences (censorship was not an issue in an old people's home) but the uncertainty about whether mail had been forgotten was similar.

What views are held by staff and others of the appropriate life-style for the elderly? Should residents be restricted like prisoners or as free as hotel guests? Should messages for residents be given to staff to be passed on to residents, as happens with most communications from official bodies?

A RESIDENT'S DAY

Mrs Richardson talked about life at The Pines and later wrote some notes about three days. She emerges as someone who is less active than some (she could only get around on crutches) but who is contented. This fuller picture of life for one resident concludes this chapter.

Nothing is boring. After lunch I come in my room and read my Bible for an hour. After tea I come in between six and seven and read the Bible again. Don't read anything else, got no time. Still sometimes mend and sew. I write letters – two or three letters – spend about three-quarters of an hour writing. About three o'clock I sleep for ten minutes. Not interested in TV. Put up with it and say nothing. Don't want them to feel 'she's up against it'. I look forward to meals to move about – not really hungry, could do without dinner – we're not really doing anything. I do butter the bread and help do some sprouts, that depends who's on. Like to feel I'm doing something.

It's mortal cold so it's easier to sit still than get up and walk around. I don't go and visit in other lounges. Do they appreciate me coming or not? So I stopped visiting though I have visited about three times. From our sitting room everyone goes to bed at eight-thirty. I have some tablets to help me go to sleep. I sleep and wake up about two or three. My leg hurts, feel it's a long time. Have some visitors, two or three one week, none the next. Still go to meetings (religious groups) in my brother's home, have done right from a girl. Religion is what makes me happy.

Mrs Richardson also wrote some notes about what she felt on three particular days.

Thursday: It's now 1.10 and I have just come back from dinner, steak and kidney pie, cabbage, potatoes, ice-cream and peaches. I was asked if I would butter some bread for tea so 3.30 I go and do it and come back again 3.55. The butter was nice and soft and made it easy. When 5 o'clock came it was tea-time so here we go again for tea. We had cold meat and chips, quite nice, and cake to finish. At 7 o'clock I go to my room and spend a quiet time alone yet not alone with my Bible. I come back again and at 8.30 go off to bed, take a sleeping tablet and when I do go to sleep I dream, some not very nice, I can't seem to get through the jobs and it worries me.

Friday: And here goes again. The lady that sits with me each day comes in for the day and has dinner and tea; so every Tuesday and Friday she sees the nurse, so in comes the nurse to give her a liver injection and back she comes again. Mr X wasn't down for breakfast and dinner so his chair was empty for breakfast and at dinner-time a Mr Y took the chair. He is a very nice man, he filled our glasses with water. He has a long walk, he comes for dinner and goes again and comes back for tea. His wife is in a home, her mind is in a bad state, he really has lots to do by the time he visits his wife and cares for the home. Most Fridays we have fish for dinner but today we had bacon and eggs for dinner and cabbage and potatoes but *we do like* the nice piece of fish fried in deep fat and some potatoes.

For tea we had a meat and egg pie, it was nice. After we had tea we came back to our room and one lady came in to say there is a man in our toilet with the door wide open. I said call the attendant and down she comes. She said: 'What are you doing in the ladies' toilet? Make haste and get out of it.' He said: 'I am sorry.' He so often does this and says the same. I have at 7 a cup of coffee and then at 8.30 off to bed.

Saturday: It is now 10.45 and a poor man of 97 tried to walk down and when he got to my seat he could not go any further, so done up. And the lady that comes in every day doesn't come in Saturdays or Sundays so he was able to sit beside me and then the attendant came and took him back in a wheelchair.

We had nice fried fish for our dinner today. I have a taxi man to take me to Moorhinch once a fortnight so I asked Matron to phone for Sunday a.m. and she has tried all day so now tonight at 7 she at last got through and I have just worried most of the day. You see he is cheap so I want to have him if I can.

Now I have just had my orange drink and 8.30 will soon be here and then off to bed. I go out early on Sunday morning at 9.45.

Chapter 7

———◆———

MR JEPSON and MRS WILLIAMS –
PICTURES OF TWO RESIDENTS

After I had completed my stay at The Pines I decided it would be useful to gather together my research notes on some residents. I selected two whom I had known well and whose personalities and responses to residential living were very different. Had I made this decision earlier the notes would have been fuller but all my interaction would have been changed.

The bulk of the material comes from brief research notes; there are shorter sections from interviews, life satisfaction tests and questionnaires completed by relatives.

MR JEPSON

October
There was a gruff mutter from the end of the corridor. When it was repeated I heard 'Open the door then'. Mr Jepson was standing outside the lavatory door on his zimmer frame and couldn't open it. I felt a bit annoyed at the brusqueness of his demand.

One lunch he pushed back his chair at the end of the meal and knocked into someone else. 'You'll have to be more careful' said one of the staff. Comments all round – one woman muttered about it, another said to me 'You have to take no notice of them, that's what I do'. The care assistant added 'They're just like children'.

While I was sitting chatting with him in his sitting area he gave me an apple. Later, when he saw a new resident being pushed past in a wheelchair, 'She's an awkward one, always being awkward' he stated.

One night I was calling numbers for bingo. Mr Jepson was playing and I heard him being told off by another resident, Mr Fothergill, for offering money (1p) for a stake to one of the women. 'You're embarrassing her' said the man. Mr Jepson was deflated and the row fizzled down.

Later that night he was one of a few residents still up watching TV after 9 o'clock. That was his regular practice, staff said.

He came out of the lift to go into breakfast and looked at the slow-moving procession of people on zimmer frames and with sticks in front of him. 'To come to this, it's strange how it happens, you're all right one day' he muttered.

At lunch he got up to go to the lavatory. He refused the offer of a wheelchair. After lunch he emerged – he had wet himself. A care assistant took him up to change him and he came back to finish his lunch. Then he sat and cried. A care assistant put her arm round him. 'It's all right' she said. A resident and cleaner nodded their heads in sympathy for him.

November

After chatting in the sitting area, he got up and on to his zimmer, he was very shaky and angry with a resident who was in his way. I thought that was because he was frightened of falling. 'Awful to be like this, awful', as he slowly went off. Later at lunch he was helped on to his chair by another resident.

December

He gave some sweets to a care assistant.

January

I was in a sitting area chatting to residents. A care assistant came in. 'Mr Jepson's being awful, he keeps ringing the bell – he wants his zip undone, wants his trousers down, wants his trousers up. Oh, I told him he'd get a kick up the arse if he didn't get on.' Other residents commented: 'You can't be on all the time'; 'He's getting worse, wants more and more done for him'. The care assistant: 'He says he can't walk now. Staff laugh at the way I talk to him but I can't be on all the time. Yesterday I kept my hand over the buzzer and he pulled his own trousers up.'

Later in his sitting area he joined in a discussion about prices. Then after offering me a sherry he talked about sudden changes in health and how awful it was.

The next day he was sitting in a downstairs room (he'd been put there because it wasn't so far for him to get to meals). Another resident was trying to cheer him up. 'I can't understand what's happened to me. Life isn't worth living. I was in the church for forty-four years but I don't believe in Jesus – he's not authentic. Why is there all this suffering? I must have been very bad.' A staff member came by and stroked his bald head. He looked round and smiled at her. Then he asked me to get a wheelchair to get him to the toilet quickly. I got him there in time.

He was sitting upstairs again the next day and rang the bell. When I went up he wanted a chair in which to go down to lunch. 'Should I take him down?' I asked the senior staff member, aware of the policy of getting him to walk. She came up and eventually there was a compromise. I helped him to get downstairs and then he had a wheelchair from the lift into the dining room. He had to go to the lavatory before he set off downstairs and again as soon as he got down. 'It's these water tablets [diuretics]' he commented.

After lunch a few days later I took him to the toilet and then to the lift in the wheelchair. He had to walk from there. I got him on to his zimmer and then he couldn't move. Others were standing round waiting to use the lift. I tried to direct the traffic, Mr Jepson fell; I put him in a wheelchair and got him back to his sitting room. He seemed all right.

He was back in the downstairs sitting room. He called me and wanted to know how I would write the report. How would I put in people's opinions when there's disagreement, say, about getting people to walk. I explained that I should put in both sides. Two care assistants came up: 'You told your son all about us last night, then.' A discussion followed, and it became clear that he had talked about being made to walk. 'We have to do what the doctor says, what Matron says, what's for your good' said one. 'You have to understand why we are doing it' said the other.

At lunch I started to push his chair up to the table. 'Bob [a resident] says I have to do it myself' he said. At the end of the meal a care assistant said: 'You go to the toilet now and you won't need a wheelchair.' I went off to the bank. Half an hour later I was back and Mr Jepson was coming back from the toilet. Two staff were talking about him. 'He had a bottle just near him and he's done it all over his trousers and shoes.' I didn't know whether he heard or not, but he stood still with his jaw set. 'I'm in hot water now' he said to me.

Then he was told to go upstairs and change. He became the focus of attention, with several staff round alternately encouraging, bantering, ignoring him.

'That other care assistant would get the chair for me' he had said. 'I don't want it all the time, just when I want to do a wee quickly.' There was a discussion about whether that was good for Mr Jepson or not. 'She'd wheel you all everywhere. Anyway she'll be back tomorrow.'

Someone else came by. 'New shoes, Mr Jepson?' 'No', said a care assistant, 'they're wet'. 'No they're not', replied Mr Jepson, and showed me his trousers (which were wet) to prove they were dry. 'Life isn't worth living' he had muttered earlier.

February

Upstairs Mr Fothergill talked about Mr Jepson. 'He's not like his brother, this one is dirty with bad manners; it only makes it worse if you talk to him.' Mr Jepson was standing nearby.

Later when trying to walk downstairs he kept saying he was stuck.

'Are there any tissues down here?' he asked a care assistant. 'Have you got some upstairs?' she replied. 'Yes, but I've not been up' said Mr Jepson. 'I'll bring some down when I come' she promised.

'Time to go to the toilet' he muttered. 'Oh I can't get up . . . it's these tablets.'

He was joking with different staff and other residents. He seemed more prepared to laugh at himself about getting up and sitting down. When he fell back into his chair I tried to help him. 'No, I've got to do it' he said.

That afternoon there was a lively conversation going on in the sitting room. They talked about their past lives, places they had all known. 'I caught the train and walked to the end of the lane. Buffalo Bill was here then', Mr Jepson joined in. (He often talked about Buffalo Bill and I was never sure to what he was referring.) 'Are you all right?' he asked someone who was whimpering with a headache. Then he talked about playing bingo and going out to the Red Cross club.

One of the staff told me about Mr Jepson's worry about his dog, Scamp, and whether it had been put down or not. 'It would break your heart to leave a pet behind' she added.

At breakfast he had been moved to a different table and he was chatting and laughing more than I had ever heard him. He would not sit in the sitting room in the chair of someone who had just died. 'He is the only one I've ever known make a fuss' said a staff member.

The next day at lunch he pushed his plate away halfway through the meal and resisted all attempts to get him to eat.

He complained to me about the effect of the tablets he was taking. 'It's not worth having them if they make you feel so rotten, I'd rather die.' After lunch he was again complaining about them, in a strange muddled conversation that I couldn't follow about going to the toilet at four and about going down the drain.

Two care assistants talked about him while having their lunch – one of them had taken him to the toilet in a wheelchair. Would another care assistant object? 'She does go on about it' was the reply. 'They're human after all. I had to leave the room this morning because I couldn't stand hearing Mrs Jones [care assistant] going on at Mr Jepson. It's awful to see him crying.'

A senior staff member talked about the possibility of getting Mr Jepson assessed at a geriatric hospital.

A group of staff were around when Mr Jepson came back to the sitting area. They were anxious to see him settled and had made him a special bag to hang from his zimmer frame to hold some of his possessions. 'Come on Ben', said someone, 'you must stand', as he was being moved from the wheelchair to his armchair. 'That's better, you can do it as well as I.' They looked around. 'Where is his this?' 'Where is his that?' they asked each other, but not him.

He was dozing when I walked past at 10.20 a.m. A few minutes later, in another sitting area, the staff came round with a trolley and morning drinks. They talked about Mr Jepson who had sworn at one of them at breakfast. 'It's getting him up in the morning' said one care assistant. 'I made him apologise' said the other. 'Well, it's a pity he swears' added a resident.

I heard Mr Jepson calling out. He wanted to go to the toilet. Someone helped me get him in to a wheelchair. He talked about his tablets being changed (though he was a bit muddled) and wanted to know if I would be around at lunch-time.

When I brought him back from the toilet a group of staff stood round Mr Jepson. He was talking about how he'd rather be a woman. 'They get treated differently' he said. 'He'd rather you helped him today than me' said the care assistant at whom he'd sworn.

Before lunch two care assistants tried to help him walk to the toilet, a distance of only 10 yards. 'You've got to walk – you've got half an hour to get into the toilet and back – doctor's orders – got to go – stand up straight – you're not going to sit down – now you're stood up – go on – one, two, that's a good boy – quiet now, Mr Jepson [*she's* shouting!] – don't ring that bell, one, two, one, two – look where you're going or you'll fall – concentrate on what you're doing.' It took him nearly half an hour, full of stops and starts, cajoling, threatening. Lunch seemed very quiet – I wondered if residents had been affected by seeing his struggle.

During the staff lunch care assistants talked about Mr Jepson. 'He keeps ringing the bell when he's in bed. He says pass the bottle when he can reach it, then he rings to put the bottle back, then rings for something else. One of the staff takes his bell away. It's much harder getting people up in the mornings now. So many need help. Mr Jepson is the biggest problem.' She recounts how at breakfast Mr Jepson had said when he saw her: 'Look who's here then, oh goodness, f—— me', to which she had replied 'Don't you swear at me'. 'I was flabbergasted' she added. They discussed how much easier it would be for staff to take residents in wheelchairs than to make them walk.

Later another care assistant said she thought he was frightened of two of the care assistants. 'He gets worried at them shouting at him, that's why he's worse today.'

That afternoon two care assistants were standing laughing. In spite of the fact that they were laughing at me, he was convinced that they were laughing at him, as he came back from the toilet. He talked about it a lot, saying to me 'They shouldn't giggle at me', and later stopped another care assistant to say 'Jill, I was coming down the corridor and they were laughing at me'.

When the drinks were taken round one care assistant said to another 'You're getting a better reception from Mr Jepson than I did'. 'I can't help it if I'm sympathetic to him' was the reply.

I took him to the toilet during lunch and he squeezed my hand afterwards.

I sat talking in his sitting area. Another resident would interrupt every now and again with 'Say "thank you"' or 'What do you say?' as I passed him his cup of tea or helped him with something. Mr Jepson talked about his time in the army, playing football for the army XI when he'd played at half-back. He had driven a truck across Luxembourg to play a match and got back to base early the next morning. Then he told me about friends he used to have in Cornwall and a nurse whom he'd met recently in hospital. She had given him a tie, and he'd promised to be the best man at her wedding, 'but I won't get there now'.

March

Mr Jepson had been taken off all tablets. He was not walking at all and was to go for day care and assessment.

I took him to the toilet. He wanted to sit there and chat – I left him and came back later.

After lunch he went to the toilet. He came back very pleased: 'I have done my job.'

I sat in his sitting room and he was one of a group that talked about rugby and a recent international.

Before lunch I sat in his sitting area and he talked about life and death and his time in the home. 'You're finished and not finished' he said. He meant that life was not worth living, he'd got nothing left and no longer believed in anything to come.

In the afternoon one of the care assistants tried to get him interested in looking at a magazine, but did not succeed. Another assistant managed to get him to walk in to meals, unusual because he nearly always had a wheelchair.

He went off to hospital for the day.

He seemed weaker on his legs; he put no weight on his frame to help move from an armchair to the wheelchair. He talked in a muddled way, not knowing where he was; he remembered getting up but then couldn't remember anything.

He again walked back from lunch, persuaded by a particular care assistant. A contrast with the day before when he did not even stand.

I told him about my car which had gone wrong. The ignition switch had not been working and he understood perfectly. Then he asked what his duties were. I talked about retirement, that someone else was doing his job. 'Who's my boss, then? Who pays me?' so I explained that Matron ran the home and that he got a pension.

Later on in the office two staff members talked about him and suggested that going off to hospital each day – a journey of several miles – unsettled him. On Friday he had come back in the ambulance and said: 'Why are you leaving me here? I want to go home.'

Mr Jepson was to be admitted to hospital for a short stay. If they could not improve anything he would return to the home and await the next hospital vacancy.

He talked very knowledgeably to me about football, he recalled his time in Luxembourg and then mentioned a court martial he had taken part in. He said later: 'I am not able to sort things out in part of my brain.'

April

Mr Jepson returned from hospital. They had not been able to do much and would take him back on a permanent basis when they had a vacancy.

    He was sleeping while I talked to other residents. Then he woke up: 'You are taking up a lot of room. How are things?' (I had been away over Easter.)

I heard an assistant shouting 'I told you not to ring that bell', and a staff member commented 'That's Mr Jepson in trouble'.

I shaved him later that day and then we talked about recent league football matches.

He told me how one of the senior staff had said he'd kept her awake all night, 'Old Nick was coming through the door with a knife to get me' he said, and got very angry with another resident who didn't know who Old Nick was. He repeated the story several times. He was worried about keeping people awake but seemed a bit happier when I said that other people got nightmares.

A resident in another sitting area complained about being woken up by Mr Jepson. 'I couldn't get back to sleep.'

A senior staff member said that she had joked with Mr Jepson and pretended that he'd woken her up.

I helped him fill in his postal vote for the local elections. He talked about politics and the local councillors: 'I don't believe in wasting votes. I've got no patience with those who grumble and don't vote.'

May

Mr Jepson was admitted to hospital. Staff recounted to me how upset he'd been, crying and asking 'What have I done wrong? Why do I have to go down the union?'

I visited him in hospital the next day and took in some clothes. He was coherent and talked about the ward but constantly returned to his question about why he had to be there. Was it because he had been naughty and been wet? He cried occasionally and asked to see one of the women staff of whom he'd been very fond.

A senior staff member went in to see him. He told her about his feelings for a care assistant at the home and how he would like to see her. He was scared he had done something wrong. 'I told him that we should keep his bed for him. I shouldn't say it, but what can you do?' she said, to me.

I arrived at the home to hear it was Mr Jepson's funeral. He was 87. Three members of staff and a resident had gone. They came back and described it as a very cold affair. 'I wish he could have stayed here' said someone. One of the residents had been in to see him at lunch-time on Tuesday and he had died soon after. A staff member commented how he had accepted the short visit to hospital for assessment but not the permanent stay.

Mr Jepson's son, aged between 50 and 60, visited his father for a quarter of an hour every day. He (the son) had decided admission to the home was necessary. 'My wife died some three years previously of cancer and it became impossible for me to keep house for an aged father and myself when his medical condition became so unpredictable.'

He had sometimes felt sad about his father's admission. 'Probably a little self-pity. A very happy family shattered by a mother dying of thrombosis, wife of cancer and father becoming degenerate.' (Probably means 'going downhill' or 'becoming confused').

He thought the best things about the home were the comfort of the furnishings, very good food, the pleasant attitude of all the staff, the opportunity of conversing with your own age-group; the worst things were the inability of all the inmates to live for each other, single bedrooms, the lack of ground-space in which to walk and being pestered by do-gooders at Christmas.

Residents were very well looked after but might profit from being fussed less by staff 'so that the inmates played a more active part in the home'. Old people should 'create a hobby and interest other people' and 'I think it would be good if some form of physical training or suitable exercises could be organised to keep inmates fitter and occupied. Not so much use of drugs but more use of the human being – less drugs – more keep-fit.'

When old he would wish to live in an old people's home 'so as to retain as much independence as possible without having to worry about my degeneration.'

This information is taken from a questionnaire completed by Mr Jepson's son.

MR JEPSON'S OWN VIEW (interview in February)

Mr Jepson had some knowledge of the home before his admission from visiting friends there. He described the day at his own home when he had been 'reading the Sunday paper and the floor came up to him'. His son had said that something must be done and had seen a doctor at the hospital.

He talked about settling in:

> I was used to the army. John and Bob [other residents] told you about things, what was expected . . . I accept discipline as it comes . . . the food is OK. I couldn't bring anything in with me [his interpretation of the policy of the home]. I would like to have brought my dog. I ask now about Scamp, and Charley [a friend who visits] says 'We let a lady have him' and I'm sure I saw him out in the street once.

Then he described a typical day:

I like getting up. Getting in and out of bed is the biggest problem, I need help to swing my legs down and up. When I get up I think here it is – breakfast – I wash my face and do my bed if I can. Everything brings back memories [he is close to tears]. My son is a good lad he'd do the utmost.

John and Bob are used to it here. They've been here years. I'm not so used to it. Look forward to going down to breakfast. She [care assistant] says 'Come on, it's eight-thirty' and I say 'I can't go any faster'. Enjoy the meals – mustn't grumble about food.

Getting to the lavatory is difficult. Sometimes I've had a bottle under my chair in the sitting room to do a wee, but Bob doesn't like it. I quite understand his attitude. He might have his daughter here.

Then I get a paper, don't read it much. I smoke a pipe sometimes but often don't feel like it. We watch TV from about four to nine-thirty or ten-thirty at night.

I don't talk much, watch what's going on up the street. Very often think 'What did you come here for?'. I try to answer the conundrum but it doesn't come off. I come up to the room with everybody asleep, there's no fun in it, though I might sleep from eleven to twelve. The atmosphere is very subdued. Nobody stands up to sing a song of sixpence. The conversations are about 'when were you born?' and 'can you remember?'. I remember as a boy keeping shop and remember seeing the real Buffalo Bill. A good many people here hold back, don't say what they have to say.

It doesn't worry me when I'm bathed. I am pleased to be able to have one. I don't get embarrassed with young ladies, they can do anything to me, got used to nurses bathing me at hospital.

Most of his other comments were to do with attitudes and anxieties.

You can't expect a man and woman to marry here. I'm fond of Sue [a care assistant] but she's married and has children. There were years and years of married life and now I'm shut up away from the world, shut up away from my family.

I'd rather lead an ordinary life if I could walk about. I've gone past anything. What worries me most is not walking, I can't get about like I used to. If I had been lucky enough for things to have gone as they should, it would be different altogether. The house up there [his old home] is a marvel, everything has been done to it.

In the army they were all one class of people – all got one aspect – here all got their own things to see to. I don't like the atmosphere much because the atmosphere is everybody for himself. If you can't look after yourself you've had it.

There's always the tendency of staff to be I'm better than you. Mrs Smith is nice. 'Anyone for any more?' she says. I don't like too much shouting. The important qualities they need are those they have at home – mucking in, having a joke. People say 'Don't take any notice of him' [Mr Jepson]. I don't like it, don't let it get on my nerves.

'Would you advise a friend to come in?' I asked. Mr Jepson replied:

I find everything puck-a-doo. I'd advise him to come in. What's the good of being in the outside world when there's somewhere to rest your weary head. The best thing is that you've got the satisfaction that you've got something to eat.

He said he had no special friends in the home, was not worried by the behaviour of other residents, thought the home should try to make people happy, help understanding between everybody.

At the end of the interview I gave a series of questions which could be scored to provide a life satisfaction scale. His score was the lowest of all residents interviewed and what follows are the questions and his responses.

(1) *What are the best things about being the age you are now?*
I very often think about when I lived in – with my people for twenty-odd years – the happiest time in my life. Sit here, nobody want 'ee, nobody got any home for 'ee. John and Bob are very good but they have got their own ties, like I have. The happiest time now is Sunday when my son brings the car down and we go for a drive.

(2) *What do you think you will be doing five years from now? How do you expect things will be different from the way they are now in your life?*
Gone altogether. I'm no coward. If I had my way I'd turn the gun on myself and forget all about it.

(3) *What is the most important thing in your life right now?*
If I knew what I do today I wouldn't be here because I'd have got married again. I'd have found somebody. My son visits every day.

(4) *How happy would you say you are right now compared with earlier periods of your life?*
I was far happier years ago.

(5) *Do you ever worry about your ability to do what people expect of you – to meet demands that people make on you?*
People don't make any demands. I get into trouble about making water in the passage.

(6) *If you could do anything you pleased, in what part of the country would you most like to live?*
In this town.

(7) *How often do you find yourself feeling lonely?*
Occasionally.

(8) *How often do you feel there is no point in living?*
Not very often.

(9) *Do you wish you could see more of your close friends than you do or would you like more time to yourself?*
I'd like to see more of my friends.

(10) *How much unhappiness would you say you find in your life today?*
When I think of the time I was married I feel unhappy.

(11) *As you get older would you say things seem to be better or worse than you thought they would be?*
Worse – when my dad was alive . . .' (sentence not finished)

(12) *How satisfied would you say you are with your life today?*
I mustn't grumble. Got no reason for complaint.

MRS WILLIAMS

September

Mrs Williams seemed the most talkative in her sitting area. She was knitting a tea-cosy. 'It fills in time', 'it's something to do', 'you've got to keep yourself going' were three of her comments. She told me that she was the oldest person in the home (it turned out she was the second-oldest). Then she talked about the problems of managing at home – burning saucepans, forgetting things. 'I decided myself to move, my son never persuaded me.' She described the problems for her son who lived 80 miles away, of having to sort out her furniture and help her move. 'They're very good to you here, you can't grumble. This is the most homely of the homes in this town.' Later she told me how she used to sit in a different sitting room. 'I didn't get on there. The staff moved me down here and sent one of the ladies away.'

A staff member confirmed that they did move people if they did not fit in a particular sitting area 'Mrs Williams wanted a lot of attention which was going to someone else. Perhaps Mrs Williams dresses better than the others.'

After lunch Mrs Williams and another resident helped dry up some glasses. (She regularly helped to dry up after lunch and sometimes after other meals.)

When the tea trolley was taken round Mrs Williams wanted some more sugar in her tea. She had another spoonful and still wanted more. 'She's had enough' said the care assistant. Mrs Williams muttered 'Oh I'll have to go to my room and get something myself'.

October

One evening she asked a neighbour who had a paper what was on TV and then decided what she wanted. She laughed away at *Some Mothers Do 'Ave 'Em* and halfway through the next programme she asked me to change it over to *Coronation Street*. A resident wandered in from a different sitting area and stood gazing. Mrs Williams looked across at another resident and raised her eyebrows to indicate 'You have to put up with them'.

Mr Fothergill had been complaining about losing a pen-knife. At lunch he told people that he had found it. Mrs Williams: 'I expect it's where you left it.' 'No, I found it in the pocket of a coat which I haven't worn for months. Somebody must have taken it and put it back.' At the end of the meal Mr Jepson bumped into someone with his chair. Mrs Williams said to me about the argument that followed: 'You have to take no notice of them, that's what I do.'

Her sitting area was very quiet without her and two others.

She went in to tea muttering about how rotten she felt – she said that she had to go to her bedroom to escape from Miss Manfield. She told Miss Carpenter (on another table) that she should have got her chair out of the way more quickly for Miss Hutchins . . . A member of staff said 'One of you can have the evening off' – Mrs Williams decided not to dry up because she did not feel well.

In the staff room two people talked about Mrs Williams. 'She's a sweet old thing but she does go on a bit. She moved away from one sitting area.' Another suggested that that was to do with Mrs Smith, crotchety about her arthritis.

In the morning Mrs Williams said she was sorry to have missed the bingo but she felt too rotten. She talked about her migraine. 'Still, we've all got something wrong' she said, as she watched someone in front of her hobbling along.

That afternoon she was in bed. I took her in a cup of tea when taking the trolley round. 'I shouldn't be having it in here, should I?'

I asked if it was all right to sit down. 'Yes, it's nice to have someone to talk to' she replied. She wanted to change some shoes and one of the staff had taken her in to the shop but the manageress was away. She talked about running out of wool for a tea-cosy she was knitting. She would wait to catch a member of staff as she came back past the sitting room. She spotted her: 'Would you get me some more wool?' The staff member agreed, though she was obviously very busy: 'Oh you are a pest.' 'Well, I know you will if you can' replied Mrs Williams.

Two days later she was proudly displaying her new pair of shoes, which had been changed. 'I'm glad to have done that.' 'You won't worry so much now, will you' said the care assistant. 'No, I was worried about them.'

She saw me and thought I did not look so well. I had a sore throat. When someone suggested taking a cup of tea in to Miss Carpenter, Mrs Williams put her finger to her lip to indicate that it was a conspiracy.

After lunch she smiled with a staff member in sympathy for Mr Jepson who was upset. Then as she helped dry up she smiled to herself. 'I have lots of laughter just noticing what goes on', as she listened to the staff chatter. When she had finished she talked to a resident, asking him how his leg was. He answered her and she said to me 'I'm the only one he talks to'.

November

I had been away on holiday and Mrs Williams welcomed me back when I went in to the sitting area. She told me about going out with some friends, and the friends she had calling today and tomorrow. She was wanting to buy a picture but it was rather difficult; perhaps she would wait till her son came. When a staff member passed she said 'I hate to trouble you'. 'Well don't' was the jocular reply. 'About those things I entered for the Help the Aged Exhibition', she went on, and they discussed how to get the entries back. Later she talked about how much she had enjoyed the home cooking when she had gone out to her friends. 'But they couldn't do it here' she added. When she talked about other residents it was as 'they', 'them', never 'we', 'us'. Mrs Draxton got up to pull the blind down to keep out the sun when Mrs Williams wanted it down and then let it up when Mrs Williams thought it should go up. Mrs Hughes found the sun glaring but said 'Better ask Mrs Williams' rather than decide to have it down.

After lunch one of the staff said to another 'I should leave those glasses for Mrs Williams to dry. She likes to do them.'

She was knitting away at a tea-cosy but rather fed up with it. 'I always do it, don't I, but there's nothing else to do.'

December

She had been out into the town and came back saying how tired she was and how cold she had got. 'I know so many people, everyone knows me, that I always have to stop and talk.' Someone had met her and given her some flowers.

Mrs Williams joined a group where someone had come to show them how to make some Christmas decorations. She was pleased that the speaker recognised her and had a chat.

She was one of a small group who went out for an evening's Christmas shopping at Woolworth's.

The next day at the handicraft group she looked round and said: 'The men let Matron down by not coming to these events.'

Just before Christmas she mentioned that all these visitors were really too much. After Mrs Richardson had talked about going to her brother's for Christmas, Mrs Williams emphasised to me that *she* had decided not to move out over Christmas, though she might go out for the day. 'As you get older you feel less like travel.' She went on to say how hard it was when people came in for such events as carol concerts. 'You see, Mr Clough, I used to come in with a group to sing to the people here.'
     Mrs Draxton turned to her and asked about bathing: 'I am sure I've missed my turn.' 'You listen out', replied Mrs Williams, 'and then you'll know if you are going to have one.'

January
One morning Mrs Williams told me she had had a bad cold, been sneezing a lot. 'Lots of people have had colds. I've got to go and have a bath – I don't want to, still I suppose I've got to, got to obey orders.' She didn't think she should have a bath when she had a cold. A few minutes later she got up and knocked on the bathroom door and said to the assistant 'Matron says it's all right for me to have a bath', and went off to get changed.

During the staff lunch one of the assistants said that Mrs Williams was 'interfering' with Mrs Draxton. Mrs Draxton had been moved to a different bedroom. The assistant had heard Mrs Williams saying 'I told you that you should say you don't want to go. Ask your daughter.' The assistant responded 'Why don't you tell Matron if you're so interested in Mrs Draxton's affairs, Mrs Williams?' To which Mrs Williams retorted: 'It's no business of yours what I say to Mrs Draxton.' 'Well it is if you are upsetting Mrs Draxton' the assistant said. Since then she had heard Mrs Williams say again 'Well, I told you you should never have gone'.

February
Mrs Williams was mending a cardigan for Mrs Richardson. Someone else had tried to mend it but not done a very good job. Mrs Williams managed it very neatly. We chatted about the weather, the snow and my son's violin practice.

Mrs Draxton called me over to ask if anything could be done to partition off the open side of the sitting area. Mrs Williams joined in the discussion about keeping the room warm.

Mrs Williams had written something for me about her day and took me into her room to read it out. She was very nervous as to whether it was good enough.

One afternoon she talked about her son who had taken her out to see a friend in hospital who had had a stroke – and she described her feelings when she realised that her ciose friend was so ill. Later she mentioned how difficult she found it when she wanted to help other residents: 'You are not to put out a hand because the staff won't let you. I know they worry that we shall both fall but it is frustrating.'

She walked past the office looking for an ear-ring she had lost. Later Mrs Richardson told me that Mrs Williams had phoned her son from the office for three nights and got no reply. Then she wrote a letter and her son phoned her that morning. 'It's nice to hear him and know he's all right' said Mrs Williams. She knitted and joined in a conversation about other residents – Mr Jepson had sworn at one of the staff – and then the conversation moved on to past incidents, such as a man who had sat and played the piano in the nude.

She said 'Hello' to a man visiting to decide if he wanted to go into the home but he was too preoccupied and didn't acknowledge her.

March

A staff member told me that Mrs Williams had asked to see the doctor about her chest and cough but had been told 'No'.

Mrs Draxton managed to complete a puzzle. Mrs Williams said, 'I couldn't do that'. 'Go on', said an assistant, 'that's for a five-year-old.'

Mrs Williams said that she usually went out to see the doctor at his surgery when her son called. I asked whether she was concerned about others overhearing. 'No, it's more that I get the feeling that the staff think I'm making a fuss' she replied.

She was apologetic that she couldn't join a group discussion because of her migraine.

April

I had been away. Mrs Williams told me she had not been so well. Her son was coming up on Thursday and she hoped to have her hair done before he came. She told me about other people who had not been well. 'I sometimes wonder about old people and what should be done. They can't all come to places like this. I used to wonder if I had done the right thing. Mrs Lippett wonders that now, but you get these moments.'

A staff member told me that an assistant had taken some tea into Mrs Williams on Sunday because she had been in bed. Mrs Williams was eating Easter cake when she went in. 'Well', said the assistant, 'if she can eat Easter cake she could be in here for tea.'

Mrs Williams and Mrs Richardson talked about someone who had had a fall. 'They say she always does that after a scene. I don't know if that's right.' Mrs Williams wanted the TV on but did not know if other people did. Mrs Richardson replied: 'Well, I have said that you have it when you want.'

After lunch a group of staff talked about Mrs Williams who must have complained about a visitor whom she knew who had come in and spoken to someone else and not her. A staff member said 'I am always very careful how I talk to her'.

'My son's like me' said Mrs Williams to me, 'always helping people. I've been helping the sick here [she lowered her voice]. We are not supposed to, you know. Some staff members would tell us not to but I can't not do anything. Mrs Roberts passed and told Mrs Williams she ought not to have gone out for an early morning walk without a hat and coat. Mrs Williams waited until she had gone and said: 'It makes me laugh all these things.'

May

Mrs Williams was sitting out in the sun when I took Miss Hutchins out. It was a lovely day and they chatted far more than I had heard them in the sitting area, although they sat next to each other.

One of the assistants came and talked to Mrs Williams about the Bath and West show that she was going to. 'She can talk, can't she' said Mrs Williams when she left. Meanwhile Miss Manfield, who was deaf, went on talking to the room at large. 'You can't tell her to shut up, can you?' Mrs Williams said. Then she looked despairingly at Mrs Draxton sleeping next to her, because she thought Mrs Draxton did not do enough.

June

Mrs Williams saw a staff member taking a doctor to see one of the other residents and tried to guess who was being visited. When Mrs Richardson said that her doctor always visited her once a month, Mrs Williams seemed jealous: 'Not once a month.' 'Yes, once a month' replied Mrs Richardson.

Mrs Williams told me that one of the staff had phoned to make an appointment for her to see the doctor when her son visited. However, it was not her own doctor who was available and she felt this other person would not take her so seriously. She added that she had been able to talk to her son on the phone in the office. She was involved in a discussion about her bath. She had been asked to get her things ready. 'Well, that must have been before ten. The assistant's not back yet and it's eleven o'clock now.' 'If you're busy I'll have it this afternoon' she said when she did see the assistant.

A few minutes later she turned to me. 'There's nothing to talk about but our aches and pains and our own small affairs. You tell us what you have been doing.' A staff member came round to talk to Mrs Williams who was said to be upset that she did not go out on a visit. It turned out that Mrs Williams had really wanted to use the opportunity to visit some people in hospital. 'Well, someone could always take you.' 'Yes, but I don't like to bother people' replied Mrs Williams.

One of the staff told me how Mrs Williams had been one of a group who went over to the pub at lunch-time.

July

This was the day an outing had been planned for all the residents. Mrs Williams was said to have gone round the day before saying 'Nobody's asked me to go' and had been told off because she must have known that everybody could go.

Mrs Draxton talked about Mrs Williams: 'Mrs Williams is a friend in a way. She's very kind to me, was very kind when I first came, but she rules me.'

MRS WILLIAMS'S VIEW (from interview)

She had been a caretaker for over twenty years in a county court. Married twice, her second husband had been at home for twenty-four years. She had lived for thirty-seven years in her house before coming into the home. She described her greatest blow as the death of her daughter at twenty-one.

She went on to talk about the decision to come into The Pines:

Things had got so difficult when I was at home. I had a home help, I had done mostly for myself. I went on and on till I couldn't cope. I was spoiling cooking utensils, letting things fall. My son never said a word, he wouldn't hurt my feelings. I wrote and told him I'd made up my mind. I had known The Pines for some time – used to come to coffee mornings.

My nieces wrote to the welfare, the doctor wrote a note for me. I'd been thinking about it for some time. The doctor said 'I'm glad you've seen sense at last'.

It got more difficult going over to see my son. I have had one or two Christmases on my own.

I saw Matron first and asked her what she thought about it [going into a home]. She sent me to the social services and then kept in touch.

Then she described coming into the home: 'I didn't know what to bring in. She, the welfare person, told me that you can take a table or rug. I sold a lot of things privately.' When she had first been in the home she had shared a room with Mrs Pinker:

I was sorry to have to move away, she was such a sweet person. I would get under the bedclothes and cough so as not to disturb her. There are times when you want a room to yourself – you've got bits of sewing or writing to do; then I had a carpet when I had a room of my own.

In the morning I came in all my furniture was gone, my son had a week off to do everything. When I came in, Matron was waiting. She asked me how I was. 'Not too bad, quite all right' I said. She showed me to my room. My son had to be back to the house. I'm one of those people that can't make a fuss. I adapt myself to new people. It was just before lunch. I knew Mrs Smith – I used to be a frequent visitor – knew several of them – I had always been pretty active.

The nights seemed difficult. 'I went and spoke to Mrs Pinker. "We are going to share a room" I said. She said "Nice to have you".'

Then we talked about a typical day.

I used to stay in bed longer, till about nine o'clock. Sometimes now I would stay in bed longer if I could. I listen to the radio from seven-thirty. It's quite easy to get dressed – I leave my room about twenty past eight. Don't like waiting before the meal, like school-children – you've got to put these things to one side. I enjoy my food. I go in the kitchen and help – help with drying and washing. Glad to think I'm here. I'm fortunate – no worry. Matron said to my son 'She's fine, she comes in the kitchen'.

At nine-thirty I go to the sitting room. I'm fond of knitting, other-wise time would seem too long. Everyone could get outside in the summer. I'm all for keeping the peace. The trouble with some people is they go too far with religion.

In the afternoon visitors may come. I sometimes go days without seeing anyone. Once a fortnight I go to the Red Cross club. Look forward to the shows we have here. The group come from the Baptist chapel. I used to sing at the chapel – you feel dreadful that people are coming in to see you.

She used to find it embarrassing to be bathed by other people but had got used to it. She couldn't get in and out of the bath on her own and hadn't been able to at home.

She said that she would advise a friend to come into the home. Her son said he was as happy as a king. ' "I couldn't bear to think of you watching the fire on cold winter nights, and then the price of food" he said.'

She thought the home should try to help everybody, though residents should help themselves as much as possible. The staff she described as wonderful and understanding.

'They won't let us help others – if they fall down, we'll fall down, the attendants say that. It's terrible to pass people and not give a hand.'

What did she like most about the home? 'I didn't like to shut myself away. I enjoy my bedroom. We can bring visitors in when we want. We can stay in or go out. I went out to parties late at night. I used to ring the bell and get in.'

She did think about what other residents said.

I was disgusted with what they were saying the other day. Amongst elderly people – don't want filth stuck down your throats.

When I was here at first Mrs Smith took everything out of my hands. She wouldn't let me do a thing; wouldn't let me show Mrs Pinker anything. It was the same at table in the beginning. 'You don't want to do that', she said, 'there's attendants to do that.' It's sad to see her like she is [crippled with arthritis]. One day I nearly ran away. 'Mrs Smith,' I said, 'have I ever done anything to offend you?' I don't worry about the behaviour of others now.

Other people I meet think this is a marvellous place, free and easy, just like home.

Mrs Williams's responses to the life satisfaction test showed her to have a score slightly above average for residents at The Pines.

(1) *What are the best things about being the age you are now?*
Having health and strength and being happy.
(2) *What do you think you will be doing five years from now?*
Will I be living? I'll be lucky if I am the same as now.
(3) *What is the most important thing in your life right now?*
To live a good life as long as I can, to do the best I can for others.

(4) How happy would you say you are right now compared with earlier periods of your life?
I'm more contented now because when I had been in the house so long I was glad to have a break, and there are no wants.

(5) Do you ever worry about your ability to do what people expect of you – to meet demands that people make on you?
No. They very often think I don't feel like I do because I'm a bit upright. In my ways I'm a bit quicker.

(6) If you could do anything you pleased, in what part of the country would you most like to live?
Exeter [her home town].

(7) How often do you find yourself feeling lonely?
I don't think I'm ever down that far. All the others [in her sitting area] do go to bed at eight, but there's something to pass the time.

(8) How often do you feel there's no point in living?
No. I've always enjoyed life – had a lot of friends.

(9) Do you wish you could see more of your close friends than you do or would you like more time to yourself?
I'd like to see more of my close friends.

(10) How much unhappiness would you say you find in your life today?
None.

(11) As you get older would you say things seem to be better or worse than you thought they would be?
Better. I can live gracefully.

(12) How satisfied would you say you are with your life today?
Quite satisfied. There are others worse off. A lot complain unnecessarily.

Chapter 8

———◆———

DEPARTURE

'Everyone in a residential unit will eventually leave it – whether it be for his family, for another unit, for a hostel, for lodgings or other forms of relatively independent living, or for the grave', writes Righton (1970), and he continues by saying that, as a consequence, one of several objectives for residential care should be 'to help each resident to prepare appropriately for departure (e.g. to ensure that an adolescent is better equipped to cope with life in his family or the world than he was on reception, or to help an old person face death with peace of mind and a sense of fulfilment)'.

Departure has very different implications, as Righton's examples illustrate, for residents who expect to live permanently in the unit than for those who expect to leave (at a particular time or for particular reasons) *and* will live elsewhere. Departure highlights the distinction between residential work with children and with adults.

An old people's home is likely to be composed of a few day visitors and a few short-stay ('holiday') residents, with the majority being permanent residents. The permanent residents may leave for a different living situation, to transfer to another residential home, to go into hospital, or at death. Davies and Duncan (1975) report the discharges from Reading residential homes for the elderly. In the period between 1970 and 1974 there were fluctuations in trends but the general picture is that about 50 per cent of residents leaving residential homes died in the home, about 37 per cent left for long-stay periods in hospital and the remainder either returned to their past homes or moved to sheltered accommodation or to some other setting.

The situation was similar at The Pines. In the period during which I was at the home there were forty-two permanent residents. These included seven people admitted during the time I was there. Of these forty-two residents: one moved to private home, four died in The Pines, three moved to hospital where they died, and six moved to hospital as short-stay patients (this includes two people who returned to the home and subsequently died in the home or hospital).

A substantial proportion of residents, nine out of forty-two, entered hospital in this period. Admissions had different significance on different occasions. For example, Mrs Hughes was admitted to hospital because she had become highly confused and paranoid. On her return to The Pines a few weeks later she was much more lively and talkative. She stated that she did not need to go into hospital but, when a staff member said 'I knew you wouldn't be gone long,' she replied 'I thought I wouldn't come back'.

Understandably this is a general fear about hospital. In those situations where a resident felt the stay in hospital would be permanent, naturally she became extremely anxious. Mr Jepson illustrates this well. He accepted day visits to a hospital, and a short stay for investigation at a local geriatric hospital. On his return the doctor indicated that his condition was chronic, not treatable, and that he should return to hospital permanently as soon as they had a bed. When he returned to the same hospital for permanent stay he was very unhappy.

The hospital was in old joint-user buildings. 'What have I done wrong? Why should I be sent to the union?' he said, crying, in hospital. In spite of the fact that the difference in the reasons for his stay from his earlier visit had not been spelt out to him, he was acutely aware of the distinctions. He died ten days later.

It was rare for departure from The Pines to be tinged with any excitement. Short-stay visitors did return, refreshed, to their own homes. Miss Brinton left, unwillingly, for a private home in which she thrived. That apart, departure meant hospital or death.

Staff were well aware of this. They cared for highly dependent residents within the home and it became too much only when they had several residents who needed maximum help, or when an individual had become totally dependent. However, that statement suggests a clarity about situations that was not often apparent.

The staff believed that residents would be happier staying, and dying, at The Pines. They knew there were times when their task became too great. They saw also that the three residents who went into hospital for permanent care all died within a few days of admission. They regretted at that stage that they had not been able to stay at The Pines. It is impossible to state whether these individuals died more quickly because of the admission to hospital. What is clear is that staff have no way of knowing how long the individual will live.

It is necessary to distinguish this situation from one where the resident appears to be dying. The staff were fully prepared to care for those residents within the home. Before looking at death in the home I shall return to the significance of hospitalisation. Acute situations create few problems for staff or residents and the decision is comparatively straightforward. The chronic situation is far more complicated. Not only are staff uncertain as to whether a particular resident ought to be admitted to hospital, the residents also are aware of the anxieties. There is no doubt that departure for hospital is seen by residents as a threat.

When the geriatrician visited Mrs Tinley at The Pines he said 'Well, you can't stay here unless you can walk', and Mrs Tinley made more effort to walk as a consequence. Mr Gasden was told by a care assistant that if he was wet so often he would have to go into hospital. When a senior staff member commented to the care assistant 'I don't think that was a very helpful thing to say', the assistant replied, 'Other senior staff members say that'. Mr Jepson did feel that he had been sent to the hospital for being naughty. At around that time a staff member had made Mrs White walk into lunch. Two residents thought she was being cruel; the staff member replied: 'What if we left her to get like Mr Jepson and she had to go into hospital, you'd say it was our fault then.'

One of the difficulties about the admission to hospital of a resident is that a bed, urgently needed by others, is left vacant. Many local authorities will keep the place for the resident for a set number of weeks (perhaps eight) if the spell in hospital is not thought to be permanent. In the meantime the room may be used for short-stay residents though the person in hospital may not be aware of this.

The rights of the absent resident do not go entirely unnoticed. When Miss Ford was in hospital, Mrs Smith told me she was sitting in Miss Ford's chair. She explained that part of the reason she was doing it was so that she could make sure no one else sat in it and that Miss Ford had it back when she came out of hospital.

Another aspect of departure was that, while in reality it was likely to be at death or for hospitalisation, for those who had not accepted the necessity of living in an old age home their dream was of returning to their own house or their family. An admission report on Mr Gasden stated that he was not going to sell his property yet because he hoped to return home and added that this was 'obviously impossible'. Some months later he still hoped to be out of The Pines, though his house was now sold.

The picture with Mrs Loosely was somewhat sadder. The following exchange took place after Mrs Loosely had been in the home about eight months, while Miss Napier had lived there for only a week or two.

MRS LOOSELY: 'You been sleeping?'
MISS NAPIER: 'No, I've been in my room, sorting out.'
MRS LOOSELY: 'Why?'
MISS NAPIER: 'I want to go home.'
MRS LOOSELY: 'Oh, we all want to do that.'

Mrs Loosely had been manipulated into staying in the home. The GP was not prepared to allow her to return to her own home and there were several instances where Mrs Loosely was told that she could not go home without the doctor's permission. Neither the doctor or the social worker was prepared to instigate proceedings for compulsory admission and so she was persuaded to stay. The result was that, always hoping to leave, she rarely enjoyed her life at The Pines. After eight months she had become resigned, though still unhappy.

Earlier the same day she had talked to Miss Napier about her own home.

MRS LOOSELY: 'I can't go home.'
MISS NAPIER: 'Why not?'
MRS LOOSELY: 'Well, my house has been sold.'
MISS NAPIER: 'Sold?'
MRS LOOSELY: 'Yes, it was a family house, you know, and had to be sold.'

In fact her house had not been sold but she had had to find an acceptable reason for not going home.

DEATH

Miller and Gwynne (1972) write of the centrality of death in institutions where adults live permanently. Institutions for the younger disabled face special problems because the residents have not lived through a normal life-span nor fulfilled the roles that are normal in society. In most other respects their examination of 'export processes' is significant for old people's homes.

Death and hospitalisation (which may lead to death) are the commonest ways of leaving the institution. In an old age home between 25 and 33 per cent are likely to die each year. Miller and Gwynne suggest that the acknowledgement of the frequency of death may be avoided; that staff may look to the nursing task rather than the individual; that little grief may be shown by staff or residents; that residents may be transferred to die off the premises. Fantasies about living outside the institution may exist and will make it 'more difficult for inmates to find support for the reality that most of them will, in fact, have to face'.

Menzies (1960) discusses the situations that create anxiety for nurses in hospitals.

Nurses are in constant contact with people who are physically ill or injured, often seriously. The recovery of patients is not certain and will not always be complete. Nursing patients who have incurable diseases is one of the nurse's most distressing tasks. Nurses are confronted with the threat and the reality of suffering and death as few lay people are. Their work involves carrying out tasks which, by ordinary standards, are distasteful, disgusting and frightening.

Staff in old people's home face some of the same anxieties. Two distinctions are important: the first is that the regular task of nurses is to care for ill people; the second is that nevertheless the typical output from a hospital is a convalescent rather than a corpse (to use Miller and Gwynne's blunt words).

At The Pines the physical aspects of dying were discussed with considerable openness. Thus a staff member would report to residents on the progress of someone who was ill, that 'she has had a good night', 'is not expected to last through the day', 'has become very thin and is dying', or whatever. There was concern to ensure that the dying person was comfortable. A member of staff might well drop in frequently to the room of the dying individual. But there were other tasks in the home that needed to be carried out and few gave much time to sitting with someone who was dying.

Residents were discouraged from calling on a dying resident. This is indicative of other staff–resident situations. Staff were anxious to maintain their control of the task and there was a feeling that residents' visiting might be a way of checking up on the staff's standard of care, or highlighting the fact that staff were not spending as much time with the particular resident as was needed.

When somebody died one of the care assistants cleaned and prepared the body and, after the relatives had visited, the undertaker would take the body away. This was usually done at a meal-time, but there was no secrecy as the coffin was taken out of the front door and could be seen by the residents.

The discussion of the death reflected the different standpoints of the speakers. The most common theme was reflection on the last episodes of an individual's life. This served the function of grappling with the inexplicability and the finality of death. It is crucial to remind oneself of the way any death serves as a reminder of our own mortality, and yet the fear of death (as indeed the fear of old age) is often hidden. There were several occasions on which different staff members commented on death in terms such as 'She wasn't any bother, was she? Always clean and nice.' Being clean was an important attribute in the staff's eyes, and a 'clean' death was a part of this. This seemed important to staff for two reasons: first, because their task had much to do with cleanliness and someone who was eneuretic or soiled herself created a lot of work for staff; more important, though, was the concern about one's own death. Staff who saw the most frail of the elderly naturally had fears as to what they themselves would be like when old and for many the greatest indignity was lack of control over one's bladder. At death people feared the final indignities of infirmity and so they wished to die without being a burden on others, and being clean, being in control to the end, seemed the most important symbol of this. In fact this is another illustration of the over-riding importance attached to the mechanical or physical aspects of dying.

Menzies suggested that in caring for the ill there were benefits and losses arising from the defence systems used by staff. The positive side of caring for the dying at The Pines was that the physical care was provided with openness, tenderness, indeed with love. Several staff seemed more prepared to show their feelings than on other occasions. Nevertheless the void that was left was huge. An institution that has up to one-third of its residents dying per year needs to confront the meaning of death for residents and staff. Residents had little opportunity to discuss feelings about the purpose of life, religion, or death. On one occasion I led a discussion with a small group of residents and these three topics were all voiced. Two staff members said to me afterwards that the discussion ought to have been about crime, sport, or the local elections.

Other residents were aware of the good physical care for those who were dying. It was very important to them as it was an indication of what treatment would be given to them when they came to die. (I am anxious to stress that by talking about 'a clean death' I do not wish to suggest a cold, antiseptic approach.) Their fears, though, like the fears of staff, had little opportunity of being voiced.

In an emotive area such as this it is never easy to know whether statements which claim freedom from anxiety about death should be interpreted as acceptance or avoidance. It would probably be fair to say that both elements exist. Some residents saw life as a burden for themselves or others and therefore did envisage death as a release. Mrs Knight talked about her 'wearisome body' and saw death as 'a good thing . . . People who are suffering and have no hope should be put out of their misery.' Several residents when asked what they expected to be doing in five years time stated: 'Dead, I hope'; 'Gone altogether'; 'Kicking up the daisies'; 'Worms will be eating me'; 'Don't expect I'll be running around then'; 'I hope to be no longer on earth'; 'I don't want to be a burden on others'. The likelihood is that most of them would be dead by then.

Mrs Knight expressed a fear of death, though not so much about her own death as of being in a room with someone who was dead. She thought this went back to her father dying suddenly when she was 14. By contrast Mr Peat called the staff one night when he thought his room-mate had died. Staff confirmed that the man was dead and would have moved the body out. Mr Peat did not want them to and was quite happy to sleep in the same room as the dead man. Another time Mrs Smith chatted from her seat to the undertaker who was carrying a coffin out, which staff thought somewhat irreverent.

Miller and Gwynne note what would be a frequent comment from other institutions: that residents do not seem to care about the death of the other – they are only anxious to put in bids for their chair or their room. Some staff at The Pines thought it callous of residents to ask for a room soon after the death of someone else, yet they expected to move residents round at table or in the sitting area if they wished. One senior staff member commented when Mr Jepson refused to sit in the chair of someone who had just died: 'He's the first person I've ever known make a fuss.'

The system allowed for little alternative. The only way one could change rooms (in particular from one of the six double rooms to a single) without other residents being moved was to take the room of a dead person. In fact at The Pines the resident who had been in the home longest and was in a double room would be allocated the vacant single room, and there was little point in any pressure, though residents may not have realised this.

Naturally residents' pictures of dying were closely related to their religious belief. Several stated that they had been church members all their lives but had given up a belief in God because of their bitterness at what had happened to them. 'How could I have been so bad as to deserve this?' said Mrs Smith, crippled with arthritis. Mrs Draxton said 'I wonder whether a person like me can go to heaven', for she saw herself as the complainer that others thought her.

A dream described by Mrs Knight was interesting. She was slowly floating away on the water, and the water relieved her pain. She woke the next morning very late and felt she had nearly died. As a result she no longer feared the moment of dying or 'passing through', but she was fearful of the 'process of dying', the events that lead up to death.

Rituals and symbols play an important part both in establishing a person's identity within the home and in acknowledging her departure. A chair, at a table or in a sitting room, and more particularly a bed are powerful symbols of the continued existence of a resident. Yet, alongside this, an agency faces extreme pressure on beds. For economic as well as welfare reasons the agency may wish to use that bed quickly. Thus when a resident is temporarily absent, usually when hospitalised, there are pressures both to keep the bed empty and to use it for someone else.

It is clear that, whether or not the absent resident knows that her room is used, to the remaining residents it is obvious. Such events are significant signs of what happens when one leaves.

When a resident was thought to be dying staff allowed her to stay in bed. In an establishment where residents had to get up each morning, this was a significant indication of someone's changed circumstances. Lying in bed through the day was a sign of illness, and continued lying in bed was an acknowledgement that someone was dying. A further indication of staff awareness of impending death was their quieter, more reverent speech and an increased tolerance when they had to wash a resident. Interestingly this existed alongside the value placed on 'a clean death'.

When a resident died staff passed the message amongst small groups of residents. Residents would see the undertaker come in to measure the body and would see the coffin leave. Staff collected money from residents and staff for some flowers at the funeral; three or four residents and staff attended the funeral. I do not know whether these people were representatives of each group (for example, the most active residents and the staff on duty) or those who had had the closest relationships with the dead person.

Temporary absence created uncertainty as to the use of a resident's room. Death of a resident indicated that an empty room and space existed. Yet there is still the need both to use that space *and* to find ways of acknowledging the past existence of a resident. The procedures for taking over a chair or bed for someone else are very important since they are the signs to a current resident of what will happen when she dies.

At The Pines dying was made harder by the resentment some felt about their poor health or unhappy circumstances, and the fears of residents and staff about their own deaths went unacknowledged.

There was dignity in the way staff responded to death and the dying. Yet there is a need also for people to have a chance to think about their fears. Indeed, the whole process of helping people to die, especially if they are lonely or unhappy, must be a fundamental task for staff in old age homes. Providing warm, physical care is a necessary stage, though only the first, in meeting this need.

Chapter 9

———◆———

I HOPE WE CAN MAKE THEM HAPPY

Staff working in old people's homes are at the centre of society's uncertainty about the purpose of such institutions. They are left to carry out a confused task in the way they think best; in addition they are left to carry a mass of feelings from a multitude of people (relatives, social workers, doctors, residents and others). They will be seen as saints ('However do you do such a job?') and as sinners ('Fancy treating her like that'). They have to live with their own frustrations when the job does not work out as they would wish. Thus different individuals will expect the home to approximate to any of the models outlined in Chapter 2. The old are to be left free but kept active, to join in with others and be left alone. The list of divergent aims could be extended. Most staff at The Pines considered the happiness of residents as their major aim. One of the difficulties that follows from striving for the happiness of residents is that happiness seems an elusive quality for many, perhaps primarily because some of the realities of the lives of residents and staff are not acknowledged.

The following passage, written by a staff member at The Pines, illustrates one of the basic realities. As was stressed in the last chapter, staff are caring for people who are most likely to leave for hospital or the grave.

Mr McNab was admitted to hospital today. I know he will be well looked after but I still find it most distressing when the ambulance comes to take the residents away from The Pines when there is very little chance of their coming back. I think Mr McNab was beyond the stage of knowing but sometimes I used to feel he had quite lucid moments. The wheel has gone full circle for him and he is now like a baby. It must be heart-breaking to see one's mother or father become like that – a hardly recognisable shell of what they once were.

This passage also shows the way in which the situation of the residents brings home to staff the realities of ageing for themselves and their families. In old age some people become incontinent, confused, bitter, or just worn out. Staff are faced with constant reminders of the harsher side of ageing.

The view of staff as 'saints' is also used to hide the fact that the job does involve tasks that 'by ordinary standards are distasteful, disgusting and frightening' (to repeat the quotation from Menzies). To this must be added the exhausting nature of the heavy physical work that is involved in constantly lifting old people. The emotional demands are exhausting as well. One of the care assistants echoed this when she said: 'Sometimes you're so tired out after a day here, trying to get people to walk and so on.'

A senior staff member described how fed up she had been on the previous day:

> Never felt so bad in all my time in work with old people. At tea there was only one other member of staff on. Mr Fothergill went out of tea, there was diarrhoea everywhere. Then Mr McNab slumped down in his chair, Mr Peat was ill, Mr Gasden said he couldn't sit there and watch Mr McNab eat, Mr Stevens was in the sitting area, spitting away, refusing to leave though three people were eating their tea in there.

In the evening she had had a phone call from one of her own relatives about one of her own family who was ill. Then she wondered whether she should have got the doctor in to Mr Fothergill yesterday, though he had insisted he did not need the doctor. Later on some other staff had been on about money, dissatisfied and grumbling away. It had all seemed too much.

In this brief picture the task entails physical care of the ill and cleaning up after them; it involves ensuring that each individual resident has as full a life as possible (and so helping to resolve tensions between them); it necessitates deciding when outside agencies need to be called in; it demands managing staff. And when, as in this situation, there are demands in the personal life of the staff member, it is not surprising that 'it all seems too much'.

In reality the work is hard and tiring, often dirty, lonely and undervalued. The failure to acknowledge this results in the creation of an unreal and, consequently, impossible task. Staff, like other people, become uncertain of values and purpose when confronted with some of the miseries of old age. Unlike others, they have to live with their uncertainties. For example, it is easy to ignore the centrality of death in the life of the institution; but to do so perpetuates a false situation.

THE STAFF PICTURE OF WORKING IN A HOME

At The Pines, when asked about the purpose of old age homes, staff stressed two objectives far more than any others. These were 'care' and 'happiness'. 'Care' was a broad term which included the following comments: 'caring for the elderly', 'taking care of old people', 'aiming to care for the varied needs of residents', 'achieving a high standard of care'. 'Happiness' was used to refer both to the home and to residents: 'trying to create a happy home', 'making a happy home for the residents', 'happy and contented residents', 'maintaining a happy, homely atmosphere'.

Most comments were about the needs of residents: 'to make the resident feel each is an individual, their happiness and well-being is the most important objective', 'promoting an active independence in the resident', 'giving each a sense of belonging'. Other responses included 'making life comfortable', 'to enrich their lives' and 'to help to die with dignity'. Thus the predominant aims stated were those that concerned the welfare of individual residents.

When asked their reasons for taking the job most staff emphasised the idea of working with people. This was expressed in terms such as 'liking' or 'enjoying' working with people. Other comments were 'liking to help', 'feeling part of a caring team' and 'helping to create a homely atmosphere'.

There is considerable consistency in the responses to questions about objectives of the home and reasons for working in an old people's home. This is important in view of the frustrations staff will be shown to have felt in carrying out their work. They had chosen a job which involved working with people, they wanted to care for them and to make them happy. They did add other reasons – the need for a job and money – but working with people was emphasised most.

Senior staff felt that care assistants' prime motivation was financial whereas theirs was vocational. Rates of pay, with care assistants getting considerable overtime pay from working at nights or weekends, were similar for assistant matrons and care staff and so it is not surprising that senior staff stressed the distinguishing aspect of attitude to the job. The answers do not provide such a clear picture. Care assistants rated financial reward more highly than senior staff but the difference was not marked. Both groups expressed similar views about their reasons for taking the job.

THE CARING TASK

At this point it is useful to consider what tasks were carried out by staff. Two descriptions of a working day follow. The first is from a care assistant:

Quite a happy day. Busy as usual. I never really feel bored as our tasks are so very varied. Tired? Yes, as the water was cold this morning. So I managed to catch up some bathing during the afternoon. Angry? No, but irritated when residents compare tablets, etc., and more or less prescribe for each other, which can cause doubts that their doctor is prescribing the correct drug for them. Pleased that Mr Jepson is having day care (I hope) at hospital. I mentioned tired not because of bathing but I think a generally busy day that keeps us on our feet. I wish that we could have a part-time care assistant for when there is only one assistant on duty various evenings. Senior staff are extremely good at helping, it is true, but they have their own work to do and it makes it very much harder for them to catch up with their own duties. I wish that residents would try and mix in socially with each other more than they do. I am glad that bingo sessions are going well. The odd resident mentioned whist drives but very few seem interested. I wonder if the League of Friends would be willing to arrange an evening occasionally – could be a small fund-raiser.

A female senior staff member wrote:

Poor Mrs Tinley sat in the lounge at 7 a.m. sleeping in her chair; it's such a long day for her. I helped her to walk to her table for breakfast; she walks quite well. Mr Jepson is still not well – I'd like the doctor's advice. Mr Gasden is better, everyone seems quite bright this morning.

Why do they always cut too much bread and butter? It's one of the things I should hate if I were a resident. Sometimes it seems harder for the staff to accept change than the resident.

The cook is not too happy about making bacon roll but is having a go. One of the care assistants spends so much time coming to the office with things for my attention, helpful most times but she can be a bit trying.

Mrs Roberts, Smith and the folk in that lounge are quite determined to get a flagpole [to hang a flag for the Jubilee celebrations]. It has given them something to aim for. I do try but never feel at ease in one of the ladies' lounges, even though they are always friendly. Mrs Tanner is sweet.

I sat on the floor enjoying the sun and had a chat with the men. Mr Peat is still very withdrawn but I feel he is happy in his own way. I asked him to go to the dentist but he really does not want to, he is happy chewing away with one tooth. Always get a laugh with Mr Murphy. Mr Fothergill has lost some of his spirit. I don't think he is so well.

Joe, my heart aches for him. [He had recently had a second leg amputated]. I wish we could do more for him, have checked his leg and think we should change his sock every day. He thinks it is better now. I must make a point of telling the night staff he needs help in the morning. I think I must watch myself or I will get too fond of Joe. I really admire his courage.

One of the Friends is busy with the ladies' hair. She really is an asset to the home. She has genuine interest in the folk.

Dinner went quite well. The residents enjoyed the bacon roll.

Mr Peters came to lunch, a timid, nervous man. How awful to get old, with no one who really cares. I hope we can make him happy. Made a cup of coffee, five minutes' peace, someone arrived to fit the office carpet. Did the Christmas club, we seem to be getting more new members. The telephone rang several times, nothing of real importance, must get the tea ready before I leave at 4. Started to water the plants – they take up quite a lot of my time, but I feel it is worthwhile, it brings me into contact with the residents.

Must do the dressing on Mrs White's foot, she is a poor little soul, I wish she would cheer up a bit.

Here is Mrs Brown full of life [senior staff member coming on duty], it will take a while to tell her all the news.

THE WORK OF A SENIOR STAFF MEMBER

Staff were asked to list and rank their ten most important tasks and indicate the importance attached to these by their senior. Senior staff listed the following as their most important tasks (the description of tasks is those of staff).

supervision of residents
being available to residents
supervision of staff
planning duty rotas
supervision of the home
planning menus
serving meals
keeping up stocks of linen
supervising residents' clothing
placing orders
commitment accounting
giving out stores
seeing to medical and nursing needs
calling in doctors
issuing tablets and medicines
assisting in the kitchen
assisting care staff

book work and letters for County Hall
domestic duties
shopping for the home or residents
running the Christmas club
looking after indoor plants
coping with any small job

While the numbers of respondents were too small to draw any firm conclusions, some suggestions emerge. One person thought County Hall staff rated book-keeping, drawing up duty rotas and menus very highly, while she gave these low priority; her main priority was supervision of the care of the residents, which she thought County Hall staff rated as least important. The only consistent factor was that all senior staff ranked serving meals as their fourth or fifth most important task. This reflected the importance attached to serving meals and the consequence was that this task carried high status. The senior staff thought it important that they served food on to the plates since they felt this ensured a high standard of cooking and presentation.

This apart, there were wide variations in the ranking of tasks. One person gave considerable emphasis to supervising stores, linen cupboard and residents' clothing – these taking five of her ten items. Another person attached more importance to making contact with residents.

Staff varied also in the extent to which they monitored the work of care assistants. Thus the morning tour of the home (or inspection) served both to check on the way care staff had carried out their work and to provide a time when senior staff were available to residents. Different members of staff gave priority to different parts. One person checked each room (including bedrooms), adjusted bedspreads, and curtains and passed through sitting rooms fairly quickly. Another spent longer chatting to residents and was less concerned about the appearance of rooms. Care staff had told her that she set a lower standard on such morning tours than other senior staff.

Bathing was another part of the work of care assistants that was open to formal inspection. Care staff had to enter in a book when each resident was bathed and if the individual needed any special attention (for awkward parts or sores, for example). Consequently senior staff would be able to ask when a particular resident was to be bathed.

Less time had to be spent by senior staff on administration since the appointment several years before of a part-time secretary. She completed most returns for County Hall, kept the account books, and dealt with most of the correspondence, including ordering of stocks. The internal administration (e.g. planning menus and staff rota) was carried out by senior staff.

Senior staff had to administer the medicine cupboard. No resident held her own drugs and so staff were responsible for giving out all drugs. This meant checking the quantity and type of drug taken by each resident, and these were distributed at the end of each meal.

Senior staff were concerned particularly about the reputation of the home both in the community and with County Hall staff. This is illustrated by an event one breakfast-time. Mr Fothergill was the dominant person on a particular table. He insisted on particular codes of conduct. On this occasion a holiday visitor was sitting at the table, and when the visitor had taken a piece of bread Mr Fothergill had removed it because he considered it had been taken at the wrong time. A senior staff member intervened, telling Mr Fothergill he was nothing but a nuisance, would not leave other people alone and *would give the place a bad name*. The staff member talked to me afterwards and was particularly angry because the visitor would leave the home and talk about what it was like. Much importance was also attached to the reputation within the social services department. Several people repeated to me that the homes adviser had said how good the home was because nothing ever went wrong and he was never called in.

The base for senior staff was the office. They drank their coffee and tea there, checked drugs and orders, and saw staff, residents, or visitors there. They would emerge from the office to carry out other tasks. As a group of senior staff seemed able to plan their work with little friction. Having completed the basic tasks, such as checking drugs, they would move on to other work according to their own interests: one person would spend time checking the stores and clothing, while another liked to administer minor nursing care, for example, helping with dressings or corn-plasters. One of the attractions would seem to be the ability to plan one's work. Nevertheless, senior staff would often be rushed; they would help care assistants, especially in the evenings with bathing or putting to bed, or would help in the kitchen if the cook was off sick, or was not working in the afternoon.

While producing the full meal for residents and staff was obviously a major burden, most senior staff appeared to enjoy occasionally making cakes. Residents would comment directly to staff on how much they had enjoyed particular cakes and the task provided both relief from some of the emotional demands and some direct satisfaction.

The emotional demands, stressed in an earlier comment from a staff member, must not be ignored. Senior staff carried the responsibility for the total life within the home. They supervised the maintenance of the buildings (including the standard of cleanliness and hygiene, ensuring necessary repairs were notified and carried out, and increasingly a responsibility for safety), the physical care of residents, staffing arrangements and all the other tasks already listed. In addition they had an over-riding responsibility which was far more nebulous, responsibility for the life-style within the unit. The responsibility for this, even at times just for ensuring the smooth running of the institution, could seem overwhelming.

THE WORK OF CARE ASSISTANTS

The care staff listed their tasks as follows.

  seeing all residents were comfortable
  getting them up
  putting them to bed
  help with dressing
  providing early morning tea
  laying tables
  serving at meals
  cleaning dishes
  taking round drinks
  toileting
  bathing
  sewing
  guiding residents around the home
  emptying commodes
  keeping residents clean and tidy
  occasional chat/talking to residents
  listening to problems
  sorting out minor problems
  bed-making
  one hundred and one extra jobs

Their work was distinguished from that of domestic workers by the emphasis on personal care of the resident. The job was officially described as follows:

Attending, under the general supervision of a matron or other supervisory staff, to the physical needs of the resident/patient involving: dressing, washing and bathing, toileting and other personal needs; serving meals and, where necessary, feeding, bed-making, care of linen and clothing; care approximating to home care of the sick. Such other duties reasonably falling within the preview of the post as may be required. (National Joint Council for Local Authority Services, 1980, on Care Assistant class I)

Care assistants, similar to senior staff, were not consistent in their rating of particular tasks. Bed-making was the task most often rated as important, followed by concern for the comfort of residents (expressed as 'seeing all the residents are comfortable' and 'keeping residents as clean and tidy as possible'). Bathing was also regularly rated highly. Serving at meals was thought the least important task by one person, while she considered senior staff thought that the most important.

One characteristic of the job is that it is basically unskilled work. (The skilled aspects include techniques of lifting, which staff may be left to learn by trial and error.) The unskilled nature of the job partly explains why there were attempts to maintain clear boundaries around the job. In a situation where the work could be carried out by other unskilled people (in particular residents or relatives), staff attempted to keep control of their own area of competence. Thus residents were not to help other residents – that was a job for care assistants. Nor should they be checking on whether other residents were all right. On one occasion a resident visited someone who was dying. Staff resented this, taking it as an implication that they were not satisfactorily carrying out their work of seeing people were comfortable. Care staff were annoyed when a domestic told a resident to put her clothes away, and the concern seemed as much related to task definition as to feeling for the unhappy resident. 'It's our job to do that' said one person.

A senior staff member expressed the attitude clearly in relation to an incident she recounted about a relative.

> The relative said to me 'I'll just take Mum off for a wash, she's a bit smelly'. Then she saw my face. 'Well, if you don't mind' she added. 'I'm sorry, I do. It's our responsibility and I've got plenty of staff to do it.'
>
> We've had trouble with visitors like that. I don't mind them doing some things but not things that are our job. *Our girls would wonder why other people were doing their own work.* (my italics)

Of course the implied criticism – of the parent being smelly – is also significant, and there were other occasions when a relative did provide some physical care: one person washed her mother's hair and another took away her aunt's clothes to be washed. However, there was thought to be a clear need to keep boundaries around the work of the care staff, arguably because it could mostly be done by anybody.

Most of the care staff had worked at the home for several years and so were well aware of what needed doing. Senior staff did check on some aspects but left the care staff free to plan their work programme. In the main, patterns were clearly enough established for there to be little disagreement. In addition the changing of shifts meant all staff understood the pressures of being on different shifts. However, there were a few occasions when people resented the tasks that were left to them. Since the negotiation was informal there were only informal remedies (discussing with other staff) unless complaint was made to senior staff.

The staff appeared to value the fact that they were left free to get on with the work. The occasional check-up by senior staff – 'why hasn't X had a bath?' – would lead to comments later about 'not being trusted to get on with the job'. It is in fact an unusual situation where the basic work with a client group is carried out by untrained workers. It is not surprising that the care staff wanted the status of their job to be maximised.

It did seem that the job provided few reliefs from the tensions of working with people. This may explain why bed-making was rated highly. There were few obstacles to carrying out the task and the result was immediate and obvious, unlike much work with people. There were not many other opportunities for relief – and none that would seem as satisfying as the cake-making of senior staff. Other tasks away from people were laundering the clothes, and preparing for and washing up after meals – both heavy tasks, probably too similar to their work as housewives to provide much pleasure. Unless care staff have some satisfying work apart from residents, tension may well build up. Gossiping provided one outlet for such tension.

Another characteristic of the work of the care assistant is its susceptibility to changing pressures. There are four parts to the work: (1) tasks that are carried out for *everybody, every day* (e.g. serving meals, taking round drinks); (2) tasks that are performed for *everybody occasionally* (e.g. changing bed-linen, bathing); (3) tasks that are carried out for *some* residents, *every* day (e.g. dressing, helping to toilet); (4) tasks that have to be performed for *some* residents *occasionally* (e.g. changing and washing a resident who is occasionally incontinent).

Tasks in categories 1 and 2 are known in advance. However, an increase in the number of residents who fell into group 3 or 4 could make a dramatic difference to the workload. For example, more residents to be dressed in the morning meant that the first call for the dependent group was likely to be earlier; more residents needing help to the toilet meant more interruptions in other work; more heavily dependent residents meant more people had to be bathed by two people instead of one. Since there was very little slack in the normal working day the pressure on staff would mount rapidly.

MALE AND FEMALE STAFF

The high percentage of female residents (about 75 per cent of the total) coupled with the very high percentage of female staff (about 90 per cent of the total) made The Pines a female-dominated institution. This was bound to have repercussions on the one full-time male member of staff (a care assistant) who complained about 'the chatter of a lot of women'. The effect on the care of residents was more significant.

The male care assistant looked after the male residents. When he was off duty the female staff would cover and care for the men. This meant that the women residents had few contacts with male staff while the men had considerably more contact with the female staff. This was increased because drinks were always brought round by women, and it was only female staff who took the night shift and consequently called people in the morning. The possibility of a mildly flirtatious relationship between male residents and female staff was ten times greater than between male staff and female residents.

Old men are less used to being without a spouse than old women and so being cared for by female staff may be particularly important. Mr Jepson wished he was married to one of the staff; Mr Gasden dreamed of being married and out of the home and revelled in the company of women staff. The women did not express similar sentiments, perhaps because they had grown accustomed to their situation, perhaps because lack of male company made dreams of husbands less likely.

Mrs Draxton listened one afternoon to other people talking about an occasion when a man had sat naked and played the piano. 'I haven't seen a naked man for I don't know how many years' she said. 'Oh I mustn't think about that', she went on, 'it upsets me too much.' Otherwise there were occasional bawdy jokes but few mentions of imagined or real relationships with men.

The dominance of women was important to Mr Jepson, who considered that women got treated better at The Pines and said that he would rather be a woman. On reflection it seemed that there was more tolerance of the frailties of women than those of men. Staff seemed to be more bossy with male residents than female. This discussion needs to be placed in the context of the comparatively little contact between male and female residents since the sitting rooms – the main living areas – were all single-sex.

Residents had companions but few friends amongst other residents. It is not clear how far they looked to staff for friendship. Certainly they valued talking to staff and they may have felt staff to be more reliable than other residents. In any case the high predominance of females – staff and residents – is again significant.

CHANGES IN THE TASK

Four of the seven care staff had transferred to The Pines on the closure of an old joint-user establishment. They had had to adapt to a smaller unit, to far less regimentation and to far more freedom for the residents. They occasionally referred to the good old days when residents were closely controlled. It would seem that the change in regime had been substantial.

There had also been a reduction in the number of hours worked. While care staff did work fewer hours, this had been particularly significant for senior staff who lived on the premises. For them, in the past, the distinction between 'on' and 'off' duty had often been blurred. Three factors were important in the separation of 'work' from 'leisure': (1) the shorter working week, (2) the demand by unions for supervisory cover for care assistants, (3) a designated member of the senior staff on duty during the working day. There had been an increase in the number of senior staff. At The Pines this had meant a rise from two to three-and-a-half full-time senior staff. In the past senior staff had often worked and been involved in the home for very long hours. Thus they might be available in their flats for consultation in the early morning or evening. The demand by unions that care staff should have a member of the senior staff 'on duty', that is, physically present, rather than 'on call' coupled with the endeavour to cut over-long hours, led to the increase in staff. The consequences were not wholly pleasing to the senior staff. One of them stated that the job was more like working in a supermarket now; they were less involved, would not necessarily even be around at illnesses or deaths because other senior staff had to be left to handle the task when they were on duty. Clearly then one of the satisfactions that had gone was an immersement in the needs of the resident group. 'On' and 'off' duty had been less significant and the job had been more of a way of life.

SATISFACTIONS OF THE WORK

Staff gave different responses when asked about the most rewarding aspects of the job. Some selected the happiness of the residents: 'to see residents happy', 'to see residents clean, comfortable and happy', 'to see the contentment and smiles of residents'. Comfort and care were also mentioned: 'to see residents well cared for and comfortable', 'making sure they are as comfortable as possible when sick or dying, relieving fears, one-to-one relationships'. Aspects of relationships were selected by two others: 'to be liked for yourself, not used', 'to feel accepted by most, that they're not afraid to approach and know I shall help with a problem'. A response that spans happiness and relationships was 'talking with residents, sharing their family life, making them laugh'. Finally, the gratitude of residents was seen as important: 'when someone says "Thank you, dear" ', and 'when you see your efforts are appreciated'.

The consideration of the dissatisfying parts of the work emphasises some of the same points. In particular the grumbling of residents, the negative side of gratitude, was frequently mentioned: 'days when you can't please however you try and people grumble', 'ungrateful residents', 'when one hears residents grumbling over a meal or over who has had a bath before someone else', 'when you are doing your best and they complain', 'ungrateful people who accept everything as their right'. One person answered 'when someone is not really happy'. The two part-time staff wrote of the frustrations of limited hours and the expectations held of them. One senior staff member thought dealing with drugs the most dissatisfying aspect of the work, while another stressed the petty quarrels and jealousies between residents.

There are some significant points in these replies. Staff valued working with people; many looked for the happiness of residents or for their gratitude; the grumbling and dissatisfaction of residents (or their unhappiness) were the factors that most staff found difficult. There is some indication that senior staff may see the tasks differently since they were less likely to look for happiness or gratitude and less likely to be dissatisfied about grumbling.

Much of the material used in this chapter is drawn from responses to the staff questionnaire. There is little that is comparable from other studies. One recent study (Peace and Harding, 1980) considered the job satisfaction of staff and the tasks carried out by staff. Staff in two different homes were asked to rate on a five-point scale their satisfaction with various aspects of the work (e.g. physical surroundings, relationships with the officer in charge). This provides a useful list of aspects of job satisfaction to be considered and shows a generally high rating. However, it does not assess the significance to staff of each item. Peace and Harding also asked staff the one aspect of the work they liked best and the predominant response was 'working with elderly people'.

A further set of questions examined the tasks of staff before and after changes in objectives in one particular home. This provides valuable information on the time spent on various functions, in particular for the larger groups of staff, care attendants and domestics. Before changes were introduced care attendants five main tasks were: (1) taking residents to the toilet; (2) helping a resident to walk or move to another room; (3) sluicing; (4) making drinks/helping with feeding/serving food; (5) washing/bathing residents. When re-tested after the changes the main tasks of care attendants were: (1) encouraging residents to do things for themselves; (2) helping a resident walk or move to another room; (3) taking residents to the toilet; (4) having a conversation with a resident; (5) making drinks/helping with feeding/serving food.

From the study at The Pines I found the expectations of staff to be a crucial factor in understanding the dynamics of an old people's home. Some of the residents will be bitter or very weary. The burden of living seems too great a struggle for some. Consequently happiness may be an unrealistic goal and the attempt to achieve it may be impossible. It is realistic to aim at making people as happy *as possible*. Unless that proviso is built in, the objective serves only to frustrate staff. Some residents will never be happy, not because of how they are treated within the home, but because of their responses to the catastrophes of life. The likelihood is that a residential home will contain a much higher proportion of this group than the population as a whole. There is a danger that staff, and care assistants in particular, see happiness and gratitude as the reward for a job well done. Yet a part of their job is to look after the ungrateful, to care for the embittered. Consequently, while understanding the importance of making people happy, staff need a broader understanding of the residents themselves. In this way a concept of the task may be built up which enables staff to consider they have done a worthwhile job even when some residents remain miserable.

Responses to questionnaires indicated a clear belief in having no favourites. I was surprised by the overwhelming response to a question which was not designed to ask whether all residents were treated the same, but which ones were *liked* best.

There were other indications of the prevailing belief. After a disagreement between two residents at a table the senior staff member moved both to different tables. One resident asked whether a person who helped her into the dining hall each day might stay. The staff member refused: 'If I move one, I move them both.' There were determined attempts to adopt standard routines for everybody. An example of this was when the drinks trolley was taken round. One resident had a cup of tea taken to her in her bedroom by some staff. They maintained a clearly expressed philosophy of doing the same for everybody – in this case tea served only in the sitting areas – while secretly breaking the rule.

There were two reasons for attempting to treat everyone alike. The first was to do with fairness – a belief that residents would feel resentful if some were treated differently from others. The second was a defence against involvement. The senior staff member quoted earlier stated that she would have to be careful or she would get too fond of Joe. There was a strong belief in emotional detachment: residents would leave and staff should not become too attached. This seems an important area for consideration by staff since the reality appears to be that staff do feel fondness for particular people and try and find ways of acknowledging this in a small way (by treating them kindly, for example), while refusing to acknowledge that everybody is not treated alike.

Other patterns of staff behaviour were apparent. One was to treat residents as children. Most people's experience of dependency is with children, their own children, or their memories of their own childhood. The temptation is to associate the physical dependence of the elderly with childishness. The consequence is that residents' feelings are treated as small matters, sometimes indulgently, sometimes abruptly.

Another aspect of this is that it is difficult to carry out basic physical caring without taking over decision-making. The most common situation where people have responsibility for bathing, toileting and feeding others is that of parents with children. It is not surprising that workers and residents, remembering the common experience of being cared for as a child, find the familiar and convenient language for toileting and feeding to be that of childhood. There may be no satisfactory substitute for residents than to talk about 'wanting to do a wee'. That only makes it more necessary to remember that the person who 'wants to do a wee' is different from the child.

Powerful memories of childhood and dependence are aroused in both worker and residents in situations where people are encouraged to eat more food, have to be washed or taken to the lavatory – therefore it is even more crucial to guard against treating the old as children. 'Do you want any more greens?' can easily become 'Eat it up then, there's a good girl'. (Clough, 1978b)

It is not the case at The Pines that residents regularly were treated as children; but it remains true that it is difficult to avoid this with dependent residents. Thus Mr Jepson, struggling to walk, was told, 'Good boy, keep it up'.

DOING THINGS FOR PEOPLE

Staff find themselves torn between conflicting expectations and may not be clear themselves as to their prime task. For example, a short-stay hospital unit for the elderly will have a clear treatment objective. Patients will be encouraged to walk and to exercise because this is part of their treatment. A long-stay old age institution is both expected to be a 'home' and to provide 'treatment' so that people do not stagnate. Relatives want to see freedom but dislike apathy. Staff enjoy doing things for residents while believing residents should do more for themselves.

Staff were asked whether they would collect something from a resident's room when a resident, who was thought fit enough to do it for herself, requested them. Nearly all staff said they would go and get it quite happily; a few stated that they would tell the resident to do it herself. The situation is comparable to that already described at admission when staff oversee most events for residents and then attempt to motivate them later.

A further question asked what tasks residents should be encouraged to carry out. Nearly all staff thought residents should be encouraged to do all the things listed which included making beds, going to the shops, helping in the kitchen, helping other residents. Where there were provisos these were about helping in the kitchen or helping other residents.

Considering how strongly residents felt *discouraged* from helping other residents, and that some thought they were not supposed to make their own beds, there seems a considerable discrepancy between the staff statements about goals and the situation as it is perceived by residents. The reasons staff expressed for encouraging residents were mostly expressed in terms of 'keeping active', 'to keep mobile and the brain active'.

The belief in keeping people active was frequently stressed. There was conflict, therefore, between doing things for people and helping them to do things for themselves. There was frequent evidence of the satisfaction staff got from helping other people. The demands on staff were changeable and would vary with the numbers who were ill, bedfast, or incontinent. Towards the end of my time at The Pines there was less pressure following deaths or hospitalisation of two or three residents. Some staff commented 'It's too quiet here now', and when pressed for elaboration they said this meant that there were not enough residents who needed help with various tasks. Yet at the time of maximum pressure staff had found it difficult to get through the work and some commented that there was no chance to talk to residents.

Perhaps what happens is that staff are uncertain about the value of their work. They can see most clearly that they are useful when they perform tasks for highly dependent people, especially as these may lead to the gratitude that staff find the most rewarding part of the job. 'You need not have done that, we'd have done it for you' said a care assistant to a resident who had just been upstairs to collect a dress. This could well lead residents to expect staff to do things for them.

However, staff did not like to see residents apathetic or lazy. 'Was Miss Carpenter asking you to get her some stamps?' a care assistant asked me over lunch. 'She is lazy, she could do that for herself.' If staff intended to produce a life-style that would support independence rather than lead to dependency then they would need to develop a changed picture of their special skills and competence. Otherwise moves towards independence would be resisted.

One of the essential factors is that staff reach an agreement on objectives. This means that the differences inherent in the models outlined in Chapter 2 must be examined. Otherwise staff pursue divergent aims and do not even hold consistently to their own aims. This results in Mr Jepson's complaint that one person took him in a wheelchair while another made him walk. What is needed is not totally consistent behaviour by staff, but general agreement on objectives, a consensus.

Another picture of staff–resident interaction is provided by the staff response to a question about the characteristics needed to carry out the job. Patience and understanding were cited most often, with several people mentioning a sense of humour. This illustrates the conception of the job as frustrating and bewildering.

Staff themselves, in answering a sentence completion exercise, stated that 'staff should not' . . . 'dictate', 'be dictatorial', 'try to control residents', 'treat residents like naughty children, especially if they are not in control of their bodies', they should not 'shout or humiliate', 'lose their temper', nor 'discuss residents' faults or complaints in front of other residents'. From what has already been written, and what follows in Chapter 10, it is apparent that all of these things did happen on occasions.

Inevitably there were occasions when I felt angry, for example, at the things that were said in public about residents. The temptation is to ascribe the blame to individual staff members without taking account of the system of which they were a part. Thus what happens is a result both of the personality of the staff member and of the system.

Some of the components of the situation in which such frustration may build up are:

uncertainty about the value and skill of one's own job;
uncertainty about the purposes of residential homes;
uncertainty about the role of the elderly;
the consequent tensions between doing things for people or en-
couraging/persuading them to do them for themselves;
the fact of being faced with the harsher side of ageing and with
death;
the heavy, physical nature of the work;
being at the centre of the tensions or guilt faced by others, especially
relatives.

It is only when some of these aspects are faced and examined that there is any hope of the job being adequately performed.

One final example highlights the problem. Mrs Black's nephew visited her at The Pines. She was quiet and he was anxious. He spoke to a senior staff member of his concern as to whether the right decision had been made about his aunt's admission, 'Couldn't staff cheer her up a bit?' he asked.

When he left the senior staff member went out of the office to talk to Mrs Black. A concert was being held in the dining room nearby. 'Would you like me to take you over?' the staff member asked. 'No, I can hear it from where I am' Mrs Black replied. The senior staff member, with the nephew's words ringing in her ears, tried to get Mrs Black to join in some singing. The staff member sang a bit, conducted, and Mrs Black sang a few words before she smiled and stopped. De-feated, the staff member moved away.

Later she said to me, 'I don't think it's what we're doing. She's ninety-two and likely to be a bit depressed.'

It is staff who are confronted by the depression or loneliness of residents. They have to live with the reality of those feelings, live with their own uncertainty about the effects of the care they provide, while at the same time they help the relatives with the guilt and uncertainty *they* feel.

Chapter 10

NORMS AND CONTROLS

Discipline is regarded as central to bringing up children but of little importance in caring for the old. How far is such a picture accurate?

'Children do not like school very much, at least in the sense that they can think of preferable activities', writes Hargreaves (1972). He argues that this is part of the reason why there is a disjunction in teacher and pupil perspectives and why discipline is a central part of a teacher's life. There are similarities with situations of group living for children, whether prestigious boarding-school or residential children's home. Staff wish to control children's behaviour at meals, to get children to bed and to get them up at set times. And staff are aware that children may wish to be doing something else and may get pleasure from group misbehaviour.

In old age homes the differences between staff and old people are not the same as those between children and caring adults. Staff are younger and fitter than the old people. More important, there is basic agreement about objectives – staff and residents say that the central task in the old age home is to care for residents. The staff provide what the residents want, though not always in the way residents may wish.

This dependence on staff is different from that of the pupil on the teacher. The pupil is dependent for good reports, good teaching and for humane treatment; the old person is dependent on services to meet her physical needs. Many residents will have adjusted their expectations of the way they should be treated. They expect to be treated as a resident of an old age home. If not defeated before admission, they may well be compliant. Another difference between children and the old is that, while both groups are aware of the effect of their behaviour on the staff, the old are probably more prepared to modify behaviour to help staff.

The situations that need to be managed are also different. While there may seem similarities between meal-times with children and adults there are also distinctions. Staff are attempting to train and socialise the children; that task is not central to work with the elderly. Thus while the old may be grouped together at a meal as may children, they are rarely managed as a group and rarely identify themselves as allies against staff. Antagonism against staff is displayed less openly.

Yet processes of control are basic to residential work with the elderly. Some examples illustrate this. First, there are tasks to be performed for or with people. At The Pines residents had to be bathed. Some residents did not wish to have a bath and staff had to find ways of getting them bathed. Even in less-structured institutions there will still be limits and tasks to be performed though they will be different. Secondly, there was the fear of the job getting out of control. The fear was that if one resident were to be taken in a wheelchair, everybody would want to be pushed in a chair. Thirdly, there is a fear that as a staff member one may reach the limits of one's patience and lose control of oneself.

THE EXERCISE OF CONTROL

The informal culture that existed amongst residents at The Pines was similar to the formal set of expectations that would have been professed by agency staff. Control is inevitably easier the closer are the formal and informal objectives. How had the expectations of what people ought to do (normative expectations) been developed?

It is useful to look at two aspects of control – rewards and sanctions – as did Lambert, Millham and Bullock (1970). They considered three facets of each: coercive, utilitarian and normative.

Coercive rewards, compelling someone to receive a prize, do not exist, for by definition the prize can no longer be termed a reward. At The Pines *coercive sanctions* did not play a major part.

Nobody at The Pines had been compulsorily admitted, though Mrs Loosely was persuaded that she had no choice and could not leave. When she wanted to go home she was told that she could not leave without her doctor's permission and she certainly did not understand that, while she was held to be at risk, she had the right to leave whenever she wished.

Within the home there was little use of physical force. Mr McNab said once to a care assistant 'Stop slapping me, you are always hitting me', but this incident seemed on the borderline between play and seriousness. Two other incidents show the way pressure on staff could lead to force. On one occasion Miss Napier was standing up stating she would not go for a bath. Having tried to persuade her over a long period the exasperated assistant wheeled a chair up to her, pushed her in and took her off. The other incident occurred when Mr Page would not eat any lunch. Usually people were free to choose what they ate, though staff would try to persuade residents to eat a little. Mr Page had not been well and staff thought he ought to eat. He would not wear his hearing aid and so the assistant could not make herself understood. She ended up by putting his bib round him and trying to push food into his unwilling mouth.

There were other coercive sanctions used as, for example, when clothes were taken away from Mrs Hughes. Of particular significance was the possibility of removal from the home. Rarely stated, there was an understanding that people who were 'off their feet' might go to hospital. This was the case with Mr Jepson and the doctor told Mrs Tinley that she must keep active or she could not stay in the home. In one instance there seemed the possibility of removal for bad behaviour. At one time Mr Fothergill felt staff were stealing his possessions and was very antagonistic towards them. Staff would enter his room only in twos so that they had witnesses of their good behaviour. Then he refused to fill in an assessment form, was told he would have to see the area social services officer when he called, and eventually came to the area officer and filled in the form. He seemed to understand that he had overstepped the mark and that his place in the home was in jeopardy.

Utilitarian processes make use of the staff control of resources. Particular residents may be allocated to sitting areas, dining tables or bedrooms that are thought to be pleasant or unpleasant either because of location or, more likely, because of the other residents in the group. The preferences of a particular resident for a special bath-time, or for particular food, may be noted or ignored. When Mrs Smith was served gravy alone for her lunch, an assistant muttered that nobody else would be allowed that. Another resource controlled by staff concerns territory. Thus staff may allow someone maximum privacy, by rarely entering her territory, or may deny her privacy.

An important aspect of utilitarian rewards is the control staff have not only of the resource but of the way the service is provided. Effectively this sees staff as a resource and so staff may reward someone by serving a meal pleasantly, by being gentle when lifting her out of the bath, by being compassionate when something has gone wrong. When Mrs Barrett was incontinent one lunch-time the care assistant reassured her that it was all right and that there was nothing to worry about. The fact that staff are able to determine the way in which they provide the service is apparent to residents and explains a large part of their dependence on staff.

The home was heavily reliant on *normative rewards and sanctions*. Lambert *et al.* state that the more dependent the individual, the more powerful is normative control. Mrs Williams knitted a tea-cosy for an exhibition and was told she had done well; a staff member told her son how happily she had settled. Mrs Pinker, who was blind, was often praised for the way she managed to get around the home. Use of this type of reward together with normative sanctions helps to establish expectations of behaviour, as when staff talked about residents in front of other residents, 'He is a nice man, that Mr Peters', said a care assistant to a group of residents, 'never any trouble, always keeps himself clean, just needs bringing out of himself.'

One of the ways in which people cope with being old is illustrated here. Deprived of valid roles, age itself becomes venerated. Miss Edwards was described as 'a wonderful old lady' and there were subsequent comments of 'she's a wonderful age'. Normative sanctions were the most commonly used sanctions in the home. Staff talking about other residents is the most obvious example of this, such as when Mr Fothergill was described as an 'evil old man'. However, there were more subtle examples. Mrs Sidney told me she would like a cup of tea instead of the coffee or squash that came round in the middle of the morning. I suggested she could get some tea-bags and make her own, either from the urn in the kitchen or the trolley. After all, in another lounge a man made Oxo. 'They'd never stop saying I was fussy' she said.

WHO CONTROLS?

Such an analysis of control at The Pines presents a part of a picture. It does not bring out clearly enough the role of residents in negotiating what happens. Residents interact with staff and each other, and in any interaction each participant takes continuing account of how the other person is responding to her. Residents try to find ways of maintaining a 'good' picture of themselves in their own and others' perceptions. Since there is some uncertainty about the value of the life available to residents (several said they wished they were dead and some staff feared the prospect of being old), the wish to be seen as a 'good' resident was more significant.

Residents consequently negotiate with staff, though not in a formal sense. They may choose to be co-operative or unco-operative when asked to go for a bath which they do not want. They may request services at awkward times. The bell rang as the staff sat down for coffee. 'Mrs White always rings the bell when she knows we are having our coffee' said a care assistant. It is even more significant that residents and staff come to agree about patterns of behaviour, though the power of staff in the negotiations must not be forgotten.

Similar negotiations took place between residents. Mrs Williams decided what television programmes should be watched in her sitting room. Mrs Edwards was a newcomer in another sitting area. She described a particular programme she liked to watch at 5.30. Miss Carpenter turned round: 'We've never had the television on at that time, not since I was here.' Mrs Edwards, somewhat forceful for a newcomer, replied 'That doesn't mean we can't have it on, does it?' and Miss Carpenter withdrew from the fray.

Staff are themselves subject to controls. Many tasks are negotiated amongst the staff group on an informal basis and some staff appear more powerful than others. There are expectations placed on them by doctors, relatives and social service staff, a process to which normative rewards and sanctions are integral.

THE ESTABLISHMENT OF NORMS

Residents and staff stated that there was only one rule in the home. This was that residents informed staff if they intended to be out at meal-times, or overnight. Though rarely mentioned, there was also a rule that there should be no smoking in bedrooms. However, concentration on these formal rules would distort the way behaviour is controlled in such a setting. The key factor is *the expectations of behaviour* that are built up within an establishment. A short list from The Pines illustrates this: residents . . . should not help other residents to move around; should be out of their bedrooms in the mornings; should not have morning or afternoon drinks taken in to them; should not bath on their own; should turn up to meals if they are in the home; should get up for breakfast; should not sit in other people's chairs in the sitting or dining rooms; should keep their bedroom tidy; should take medication prescribed for them; should bath when requested.

These were general expectations, which would have been accepted as normal practice within the home. Individual residents had additional ideas of expectations or of variations on the above. Mrs Smith said that staff liked them to be out of their rooms and to eat a lot at meals; Mrs Richardson that she would like to make her bed but was not allowed to; she said also that staff did not like you to ring the bells at night, and that residents should be grateful for the help they received. In this way individuals construct their own set of norms or expectations. At times one person believed there were expectations which were at direct variance with those which senior staff thought to exist. Sometimes these were established as a result of misinterpretations – one resident might pass on inaccurate information to another. However, there were times when care staff, for example, stopped someone going into her bedroom in the afternoon, perhaps because they wanted to keep an eye on her; or complained, as Mrs Richardson overheard, about the night bell being rung. Seemingly small incidents build up into powerful pictures for residents of what they may and may not do. There may be few formal rules but behaviour may still be circumscribed.

An example of such circumscribed behaviour relates to relationships between men and women. It has already been noted that men and women sat in separate lounges. Originally this would have resulted from the strict segregation in the old institution and the design of the new building. Sitting areas 3, 4, 5 and 6 had bedrooms near them. The obvious pattern was for the residents who had particular bedrooms to use the nearest sitting area. Originally sitting area 4 had been a men's sitting area, with men's bedrooms leading off. There had been a small fire in a waste paper basket some years earlier and it had been decided to transfer the men to sitting area 1, though they continued to use some of the bedrooms adjoining sitting area 4. The only opportunity for men and women to meet was at meals (some tables were mixed though residents did not choose where they sat), at special events and if one resident visited another in a sitting area. Residents rarely visited others in different sitting areas, though people might stop for a short chat as they passed by. With little visiting of any sort there was little likelihood of men and women visiting each other.

In addition there appears to have been some control of behaviour at meals, the one formal occasion when men and women might meet. I was told that a man and woman who sat together at meals had grown fond of each other and had held hands at the table and that a senior staff member had transferred them to other tables. Whatever had happened, some people understood such relationships to be prohibited. Again there were no rules about such a code of conduct but the results were just as pervasive.

It has already been mentioned that different individuals responded to such norms in different ways. Mr Arthur and Miss Tippett did not leave their bedrooms in the morning; Mr Stevens would not get up if he did not wish to. Therefore, if one was prepared to ignore the norms, staff found it difficult to enforce them. They labelled the individual stubborn or confused, left her alone and maintained the norm for everybody else. This reinforces the earlier statement about the power of normative control increasing with the dependence of the resident. Those very few residents who regularly flaunted conventions were physically fitter than most others but, more crucial, lived more separate lives. They were less dependent on interaction with others.

By contrast, Mrs Draxton was very worried about keeping her room tidy; Miss Brinton was frightened 'for her life' of being late for meals; Mr Murphy wore a tie every day though he disliked wearing it.

THE STAFF ROLE

The more services staff provide, or the more they do for residents, the more power they have over their lives. Residents are dependent on staff for the provision of most basic services – food, drink, warmth, laundering of clothes, bathing; some residents are dependent for much more – help with getting up and getting to bed, getting to the toilet or in to meals. As already stated, staff may be kind or miserable, efficient or inefficient in the way they act when meeting needs.

Staff serve also as powerful models and authority figures. Various comments about a senior staff member illustrate this. On one occasion Mrs Sidney did not attend a club meeting, though the transport came to collect her. 'I thought she [senior staff member] would be angry but she wasn't. Perhaps she understood because she had a cold as well.' Miss Carpenter decided not to go on an outing: 'She [senior staff member] was very good about it.' Mrs Quigley related how the senior staff member had been cross that she had thrown some bread out on to the lawn for the birds.

In addition staff take on the task of supervising what goes on between residents. When an argument developed in the dining hall a care assistant moved across to control it. Both they and the residents expected them to do this. The tendency was for staff also to initiate conversations, though this was by no means invariable.

The fact of being a resident also led to an assumption on the part of many people that communications should be made with the staff and not with the resident. Details of hospital appointments were sent to the senior staff; the arrangements for the transport home of a holiday visitor were made with the secretary. Several residents wished to have a large flagpole erected on which they could fly a huge Union Jack for the Jubilee celebrations. The council official who called to explain that such a request needed planning permission which would take too long to be granted spoke to senior staff, not to the residents who had written to him.

CONTROL OF LIFE-STYLE

The extent to which residents have control of their life-style is an important variable in analysis of residential living. Some residents are highly dependent on others for the meeting of physical needs while nearly all residents have most basic services carried out for them. If residents are to feel freer to assert themselves against the norms of others they must establish greater mastery of their lives. There are three possible approaches.

The first is to consider whether staff need to provide all the services they do. An obvious example at The Pines is the drinks taken round mid-morning and mid-afternoon. Could some residents make their own drinks? If that were thought impossible, would it be beneficial for residents to serve themselves, and each other, from a trolley? Staff took between thirty and forty-five minutes to take round the trolley, so considerable staff time might be saved. However, this did create a situation where some discussion took place between staff and residents but it would be possible to allow this to happen in other ways. A development of this would be to encourage relatives to share more in running the home. An example of this is discussed by Pain (1973). She writes about a small home that expects relatives to give one day's work per week towards running the establishment. It is suggested that this improves the relationships between relatives and the old person in the residential home. The contention here is that residents would be more free to behave as they wish if they were less dependent for all services on staff.

Secondly, there are situations where residents will continue to need substantial help. A heavy, handicapped person will need to be bathed by staff who are skilled in lifting or using special aids. It is still possible for the resident to have some control over what happens. This may be by finding out *the time* at which she likes to be bathed; by asking her *the way* in which she enjoys being bathed or the clothes that she would like to wear afterwards. It is the start of an attempt to ensure that the resident continues to plan for herself.

Thirdly, there are formal ways of involving residents. The Friends (a group of voluntary helpers) had decided to spend some money raised for the home on an electronic organ. Some residents who did not want the organ thought they ought to be involved in deciding how money was spent for them. A start had been made at The Pines by appointing a resident to the Friends' committee where she could make known the views of other residents.

FREEDOM WITHIN LIMITS

The Pines is an example of a home with few formal constraints. Residents and relatives both valued the fact that the latter could call in at any time without seeing staff; both groups were pleased that residents were free to come and go as they wished. Nevertheless, the processes of control were powerful, and normative rewards and sanctions were particularly influential, because of the number of services staff carried out for residents. Control processes were also subtle. Care staff took round an early morning cup of tea to each resident and called back about half an hour later to collect the cups; this allowed them to check whether residents were getting up. Sometimes the processes were direct: 'Wakey wakey, Mrs White. I'm told that every time I see you sleeping I've got to wake you up. If you sleep in the day-time you won't sleep at night' said a care assistant. And sometimes the normative sanctions used were frighteningly powerful. Miss Manfield, who was blind and substantially deaf, had been in an argument at lunch-time.

By the end of the meal she was in tears and she told me her version of the story as I took her back to her room.

They asked me if I wanted any more lunch. I said 'No there wasn't any meat in what I had'. It's happened before with bacon and tomatoes that I had no tomatoes, only juice, or with steak and kidney. The senior staff member says she serves dinners so she knows there is meat but I say they must have given it to the wrong person. Just because I'm blind doesn't mean I don't know what I'm eating.
She [senior staff member] called me a 'miserable old woman', she shouldn't say that in front of everyone. I love her dearly but she shouldn't say that in front of everyone.

Encapsulated in this episode are dependence and love, power and control. Miss Manfield was often grumpy and awkward, she was not an easy person to have around and she might complain a lot. Whatever the reasons that make understandable the staff reaction of calling her 'a miserable old woman', the immense control from the use of that sanction cannot be ignored.

Chapter 11

AGEING IN THE INSTITUTION

Mr Jepson stood one morning outside the lift, looked at the group of people moving slowly along to breakfast, and said: 'To come to this.' He was confronted with a visible reminder of his present state by this picture of other people. It is not possible to separate out his feelings about living in a home from those about being old. The likelihood is that both were significant factors. It is this interplay between living-style and ageing that is the focus of this chapter.

THE STUDY OF AGEING

Gerontology, the study of the processes of growing old, has examined many questions. What happens as people get older? Is ageing inevitable? Is there a way to combat ageing? Are some patterns of ageing more successful than others? How significant is personality in ageing? How far do social and cultural factors influence the way people age?

One way to start the consideration of these issues is with the physical aspects of ageing. Brain cells are lost and not replaced, though it is clear that the process affects individuals in different ways. It is only (so far!) in the realm of science fiction that this process can be halted. Most other cells are replaced but with some loss or error. The effects of this are discussed by Puner (1974). The individual

> is less sensitive to touch and pain, has reduced sense of hearing, smell and taste; has a lower body temperature; has problems in digestion; is faced with less efficient circulation and breathing (heart does not pump as much blood, lungs no longer have the same capacity); has slower voluntary movements; will have less elastic and drier skin, hair will turn white; will have 'a stooped and shuffling gait' as a result of the stiffening of joints and decalcification of the bones; will have weaker muscles and will also be shorter and lighter.

The process of ageing is a gradual one and is a part of the total life-cycle. For the young child ageing means growing, getting stronger and more skilful, developing her intelligence. These progress at different rates. Thus physical size may be reached before 20, while strength and skill reach their peak between 25 and 30. The significance of this is that adults *for most of their lives* (after 35 or 40 certainly) have to get used to a decrease in physical performance. For most this would seem to be acceptable because it is not sudden and because the life-style typically expected of the mature adult does not demand high performance of physical strength. The individual continues to cope while she has the resources (in this case physical ability) to meet the expectations placed on her.

The decline in physical performance becomes less acceptable when it becomes more sudden and when the individual can no longer meet expectations. For many this occurs not at retirement age but between 70 and 80. It is at this age that chronic problems increasingly take their toll. Medicine seems better able to treat acute conditions than chronic. Thus the old are kept alive but long-term illnesses remain – rheumatoid arthritis, bronchitis, strokes, cancers – together with bodily changes that lead to daily living problems, for example, susceptibility to falls or incontinence.

In addition the brain may suffer irreversible physical damage, perhaps described best as neuronal degeneration since the common phrase 'senile dementia' is used haphazardly. As with other forms of mental illness there is uncertainty about much diagnosis – when is confusion the result of deprivation in the social situation, when caused by side-effects of medication and when the result of an early stage of neuronal degeneration?

Intellectual capacity is an important aspect of this discussion. A part of the reason why the adult usually adapts successfully to a decline in physical strength is that intellectual performance does not decline at the same rate. Puner (1974) discusses this in relation to output and has examples of both young and old who have made significant contributions to thinking or creativity. However he makes the point that while those of 60 plus may have developed skills *in the methods* of creating change, they may be more limited in the types of solutions they are prepared to consider.

Chown (1972) divides the psychological aspects of ageing into two parts – cognition and personality. The first of these includes variations in intelligence, the factors that influence it, learning and memory; the second part takes account of the effect growing old has on personality – the key question becomes 'how do people adapt in old age?'. Some variations with ageing can be demonstrated – for example, short-term memory is less effective and old people find it harder to transmit items to their long-term memory. However, if distracting information is removed and the old are given guidance into ways of linking ideas to aid memory, their capacity to remember can be improved considerably.

The effect of ageing on personality needs to take account of the social setting. The social problems of the old have been detailed in many places – typically the old have stopped working (often compulsorily) and are deprived of their position in society as workers; they may be bored; they are some of the poorest members of society while in increasing need of services; friends, relatives and spouse may have died; housing may no longer be suitable.

The picture of the old as purposeless and role-less has some truth but demands certain provisos. There is a danger of picturing a mythical past when the old were cared for in loving families. All the evidence points to families continuing to care, often at great cost, and the pictures of the past ignore the struggle and work that was demanded from most old people until they died. Today many of those over 60, with labour-saving gadgets and pensions, may not know what to do with their time. In the past, by and large, people had not such freedom of choice; they had to work to survive.

The social and physical aspects of ageing do affect personality. It has sometimes been suggested that those who enter institutions in old age have dependent personalities. Tobin and Lieberman (1976) find no evidence for this. Their case study of Mrs A. illustrates the ways in which people's needs and attitudes change.

> She was described by the interviewer as extremely friendly, outgoing, warm, pleasant and alert. Aged 77, she had suffered from the effects of a stroke, but had decided, after her husband's death a year before, not to go into an old age home. Her family had discussed this but helped her find an apartment when they understood that was what she wanted. However, her sister died and Mrs A. had to undergo further surgery which necessitated convalescence. She decided to apply for admission to a home. It appears to have been 'an accumulation of events that overtaxed the strong residual capacity', since the sister's death and the further surgery occurred only a year after her husband's death. While it was stated that 'there was a certain amount of realism in her expectations about her future in the home . . . adverse changes were noted in three areas from pre- to post-application: cognition, affective responsiveness, emotional life, particularly with respect to anxiety and depression'. Thus particular events led to changes in attitudes.

'Ageing in the institution' must be examined as part of this wider picture of 'ageing in society'. When the latter is neglected the institution is held accountable for factors that should be attributable to ageing. In their eighties people in whatever setting have to adapt to loss of mobility, to failing ability to manage housework and to the accumulation of losses. Daily living may become burdensome; there may seem to be nothing to do and too much time in which to do it.

AGEING IN PROSPECT

Tobin and Lieberman make it clear that behaviour in institutions cannot be understood solely by looking at what happens within the institution. Events that precede entry to the institution are also significant and in particular people adapt their behaviour during the period after accepting admission to a home and before going in – Tobin and Lieberman call this 'anticipatory institutionalization'.

If residential institutions were highly regarded, anticipation of the event would have the opposite result. In fact, going into a home is, in itself, often regarded as a sign of failure. Thus Goldberg (1970) considered ways of evaluating field social work with the aged and considered that entering a residential home was a sign of failure. Probably most people would regard the admission to a home of their parents or themselves as an indication of failure, whether of themselves or of the caring-system. The old age establishment, like many other residential establishments, is caught in a double bind. Its very existence is a demonstration of unsuccessful ageing, while inside it is supposed to be able to produce happy and contented people.

The view held of a home is not formed by an old person in a vacuum. The interaction between the opinions of an individual and of others in the community is important. For this reason part of my study was to find out the feelings of professionals working with the elderly and of relatives, because both groups have a significant influence on attitudes to ageing and residential homes.

Most respondents professed a highly positive attitude to old age. Table 11.1 shows the replies given to a series of statements about old age. Of forty-five respondents, twelve were field social workers and administrators, ten were nurses in a geriatric hospital or health visitors, nine were staff from The Pines, six were general practitioners, five were relatives and three were lay people interested in the home (two members of the Friends, one local councillor). Some respondents did not answer all questions, so the total number of responses to each statement does not total forty-five.

Some clusterings of responses emerge. Old age was not seen as the dreariest time of life. It was regarded as a time when one had opportunities to do new things. The old were not seen as having boring lives, nor did they make people feel depressed. It was thought possible to be as happy when one was old as when young. Significantly, activity was rated highly – the old were thought happiest when they

Table 11.1 *Statements about old age*

Statements	Responses		
	Agree	Disagree	Don't know
(1) Old age is the dreariest time of life	8	26	10
(2) Old age provides an opportunity to do things you've never had time for before	28	9	6
(3) It's a young person's world	16	20	7
(4) Families don't care about old people as they used to	19	20	5
(5) Old people are best off in their own homes	29	5	9
(6) It is better to keep on working till you drop	10	27	7
(7) Old people have boring lives	7	25	11
(8) Old people make one feel depressed	7	30	8
(9) Old people should retire earlier to make way for the younger	14	15	13
(10) You can be as happy when you're old as when you are young	33	5	5
(11) More money ought to be spent on keeping people out of residential homes	32	6	5
(12) Old people are happiest when they have plenty to do	37	1	6
(13) Old people can generally solve problems better because they have more experience	10	23	10
(14) The happiest old people are those who expect to see fewer people and to do less as they age	13	21	10

had plenty to do. There was strong support for spending money to keep people out of residential homes, and for regarding the old as best off when in their own homes. Other statements had more mixed responses.

Numbers of respondents from any work-group were small, so the following analysis provides hints not conclusions. Staff from the home and field social workers were nearly unanimous in viewing old age as an opportunity, and made few negative statements. Nurses were only slightly less positive. However doctors (a small group of six) took a more negative attitude. Four thought old age dreary, three did not think of old age as an opportunity. It is interesting, too, that three of the six who thought it better to keep on working till you drop were doctors (none were social workers), and doctors were strongly opposed to the idea of early retirement, whereas other groups were divided.

There are several questions from this. Do doctors see more of the very frail old and is their negative attitude realistic? Are social workers professing a current respect for old age which does not match up with what life is like for many of their clients? Are the differences to do with different types of personality entering different professions?

The views of those who work with old people are significant because of the way in which they may transmit attitudes to relatives, the elderly themselves, or other professionals. Many of the answers to the question 'What do you look forward to most about being old?' stressed the opportunity for hobbies and reading. 'Time' was frequently mentioned – 'time for *me*', 'time to read', 'time to do all one's wanted', 'time to choose', 'spare time', 'time to be with my wife/husband'. It is the fact of not working that is seen as providing significant opportunities, for some people, to be with family or grandchildren. There are two points here. First, a part of looking forward to old age is to do with hanging on to dreams. The hope is that this will be the time when a person really gets down to all those things she has intended to do. Secondly, this picture is built up on the belief that people will have the resources of health to carry them through. Some people at The Pines were particularly bitter that their dream of 'time to do things' had been shattered by illness. The fact remains that in prospect the early years of old age are seen as providing freedom from routine and a measure of 'living for self'.

This highlights some important considerations about old age. It represents freedom from the constraints which typify much of life – caring for a family and work. It is the early years of old age to which people look forward, though one-fifth of respondents stated that they looked forward to 'nothing' in old age. In fact there are constraints for the old, such as lack of resources or the limitations imposed by the expectations of others. In addition, giving up work may deprive people of status and meeting friends.

By contrast the fears expressed by respondents about old age refer to situations which occur most usually to the old old. In many replies there was considerable feeling, not surprising in a group of people who worked with the most ill or handicapped elderly. The most frequent fear was expressed as 'loss of independence' or 'becoming too dependent on others' (ten responses). In similar vein were answers which specified 'not able to look after self' (seven responses), 'incapacity' (five responses), 'helplessness' (two responses), with several more specifying varieties of physical disability: 'crippled', 'unable to walk', 'blindness', 'loss of senses'. Five people mentioned 'mental impairment' or 'senility'. A further two people wrote about incontinence, with others mentioning 'being ill', 'chronic illness', 'steady deterioration'.

It is clear that the major fear of respondents was that they might become unable to look after themselves and consequently dependent on others. In fact thirty-six people mentioned this. A small group (nine) were concerned primarily with their position in society – 'becoming discarded', 'uselessness', 'being a nuisance', 'not being cared for', 'loneliness', 'being a burden', 'taken over and managed like a child'. Only one person said she dreaded nothing and one other said she did not want to become bitter. The most powerful statements came from relatives of old people at The Pines, perhaps because it was hard to come to terms with the reality of ageing for someone known to you. One of these fears was expressed as 'becoming incontinent and degenerate without the courage to end it all'.

The picture of old age held by those working closely with the old is of great significance in respect of the expectations they held about performance and behaviour. To recapitulate: they saw old age as a time of opportunities, in particular for hobbies, as a period of freedom from constraints; they dreaded becoming dependent. The beliefs about what old people ought to do are tied closely to these expectations. The statement that got the most support (see Table 11.1) was that old people are happiest when they have plenty to do. This was echoed in the responses to a sentence completion exercise. 'Residents ought to . . . '

> be kept occupied where possible;
> try to keep mobile;
> appear to have more to do;
> live as full a life as possible;
> be encouraged to do more in a day;
> be more active.

These were examples of a very clear picture that residents ought to do more. It was echoed in other places. Respondents were asked to state how a resident, who was thought able to walk but did not wish to, should be treated. The overwhelming answer was that there should be gentle encouragement. Most respondents also thought that a resident who wished to stay in bed in the mornings should *not* be allowed to; it should be noted that this question did produce a wider spread, with some people stating: 'Why not, after a busy life?' The idea of disengagement being satisfying was much less common. For example, only eight people (out of forty-five) mentioned 'tranquillity and contentment', 'being at peace', 'things in perspective', 'acceptance', 'not caring', as factors they looked forward to in old age.

Old age in the future offers the hope of dreams to be fulfilled. Most dreams appear to be of things we want to do – that is, new activities. Yet the older one gets, the more one is forced to accept that certain things cannot now be accomplished. Erikson (1950) writes:

The lack or loss of this accrued ego integration is signified by fear of death: the one and only life-cycle is not accepted as the ultimate of life. Despair expresses the feeling that the time is now short, too short for the attempt to start another life and to try out alternate roads to integrity.

The onlooker is faced with his dreams for the future, together with the uncertainty about the purpose and value of life that old age makes explicit. His expectations of his own 'young old age' (60–75) are transferred to the 'old old' (80-plus). It is at this point that the expectations and fears of different groups merge.

FEELINGS ABOUT RESIDENTIAL LIVING

Another aspect of these expectations concerns the prospect of life in a residential home. Most residents stated they would advise other old people to live in a residential home, though some provisos were added. It may be argued that this was a defence, that they needed to see living in a home as a satisfactory way of life. However, the provisos and other comments would seem to allow for slightly different explanation. Living in a residential home was not the preferred lifestyle. Nevertheless, *given their present circumstances* it was the best available situation.

The group of outsiders were not keen on the prospect of life in a home. About 30 per cent stated they would consider a residential home for their parents when old, while slightly more, 36 per cent, would consider a home for themselves. The major reasons for considering a home were either that people did not wish to be a burden on children or that they were incapable of looking after themselves. Typical of this response was the person who stated that she would not wish to go into a home from choice 'but – yes, if unable to take care of self – certainly rather than live with my children, even though we have a happy relationship'. Those who did not wish to see themselves or their parents in an old people's home gave one of two main reasons: that families should care for the elderly or that they valued independence too highly. They mentioned also loss of privacy and choice, loss of individuality, that parents would have hated it, or their parents were not suited to communal living. A woman whose mother was in The Pines said that she herself would not wish to live in a home because she did not wish to be old and helpless. This statement captures much of the image held about residential life.

Other questions asked what people would like or dislike most about residential living (not about living at a particular home; see Table 11.2). The worst aspect of residential living was thought to be *lack of privacy.* Thirty per cent of respondents thought this the single worst aspect while a further 18 per cent placed it lower down a list. 'The lack of real privacy from staff and inquisitive residents' was how one person expressed it.

The other main areas of dislike were the loss of independence, regimentation, the other residents and having few of one's own possessions. It was not always clear to what the loss of *independence* refers – in some instances it seems to be loss due solely to ageing or handicap, in other cases it refers clearly to the system of residential living, for example, 'being dependent even for light refreshments'.

Table 11.2 *Factors rated 'best' and 'worst' aspects of residential life*

	Best	
	Staff	*Outsiders*
(1)	Comfort and warmth	Freedom from worries
(2)	Meals	Company
(3)	Companionship	Security
(4)	Freedom from worries	Comfort
(5)	Security	Meals
(6)	Something going on	Something going on
	Worst	
(1)	Communal feeding	Lack of privacy
(2)	Routine	Regimentation
(3)	Shared bedrooms	Dependency
(4)	Dependency	Other residents
(5)	Lack of privacy	Few personal possessions
(6)	Other residents	Boredom

Under the heading *regimentation*, I have grouped comments that refer either to routines or to staff control. Such statements were: 'being told what to do', 'the loss of the ability to decide when and how', 'bossy and officious staff', 'unwavering timetables', 'regular meal-times', 'daily bath', 'adapting to routine', 'fixed times for activities', 'institutional cooking', 'early to bed', 'a bit too clinical', 'no cups of tea when I want to', 'limited choice of menu'.

The heading *other residents* is used to refer to the factors that were disliked about living with others. Dislikes were: 'sharing a bedroom', 'other people and their funny ways', 'living with people not chosen or liking', 'the attitude of some residents', 'being interrupted when I am reading or writing', 'the difficulty of escaping from undesired company', 'other residents sitting around', 'mixing only with old people'.

There was apprehension also about *being without familiar possessions.* This was referred to as 'the loss of home surroundings', 'the loss of possessions', 'not having one's own furniture', 'not my own home or garden'.

Other comments referred to communal living: 'being treated like a child', 'having no visitors to sleep'. A small group wrote about 'boredom', 'no responsibility', 'inactivity', 'lack of occupation', 'too little to look forward to', 'being cabbages', 'lack of intellectual stimulus'.

There was a wide scatter of answers between professional, age and sex groupings. There were two slight clusterings: first, social workers disliked lack of privacy more than other groups; secondly, 40- to 50-year-olds were most apprehensive about routine and regimentation, with lack of privacy as a second concern, while 50- to 60-year-olds reversed this – they saw lack of privacy as the worst factor with routine as the next worst. Numbers are too small to be significant but it may be that a larger study would bear out that as people get nearer to the age of retirement they are more concerned about being able to withdraw than about being organised.

The best parts of residential living were thought to be freedom from responsibilities and wants, comfort and warmth, meals, companionship, security, something going on.

Freedom from responsibilities and worries was thought the best aspect of residential living and in particular referred to freedom from financial worries ('relief from bills'). In addition it included not having to care for oneself, 'being free from chores and housework', 'no responsibility for household maintenance'; 50- to 60-year-olds included this response more than any other group which suggests that people nearing retirement look forward to a time when they are free from worries.

Warmth and comfort needs little elaboration but is realistic in terms of the struggle to keep warm faced by many old people.

Companionship is the other side of the coin to the feelings about living with people you dislike: 'the possibility of companionship', 'company when required', 'relationships with good staff and pleasant residents', 'stimulation of company'. Younger age-groups were more likely to mention this item.

They were less likely to mention *regular and well-balanced meals*. While only one person thought this the best aspect of residential living, it was regularly mentioned lower down the list.

The word *security* was often written without elaboration. However, for several respondents it meant 'not being alone at time of crisis', 'always someone to hand should I fall'.

Finally the last heading: *something going on*. Specific comments were made about 'organised entertainment', 'participating in organised activities and services', 'stimulating interests'.

Other aspects that were mentioned less frequently were: 'understanding and kindly care of staff', 'time to do other things', 'being cared for' (slightly different from 'freedom from responsibilities'), 'not being a burden on one's family', 'not feeling unwanted'.

Doctors rated warmth and security more highly than did other groups. This may well have to do with the problems of ageing that they witness.

Relatives were the only group to mention constant attention and several rated this as the best aspect of living in a residential home. This would seem linked to their own anxieties about relatives and their consequent relief that their relative now had constant attention. However, the more substantial differences were between the staff and outsiders.

ACTIVITY AND THE STOP-GO REGIME

The picture of residential living that was held by those who were not residents is reinforced from other parts of the questionnaire. Answers to sentence completion exercises showed that respondents thought that residents ought to be more active, do more and share in decision-making; the most frequent comments about staff were that they should not drill or be bossy, over-protect, impose their own preferences, talk to the old as if they were children.

The predominant belief of outsiders was that to be happy in old age people needed to keep going and doing things. It has already been shown that the same was true of staff. The belief was particularly influential when coupled with that of a professional system – as when doctors looked towards treatment and cure, social workers towards treatment and growth.

In addition most residents believed in an activity model of ageing. At the same time there were residents who were physically unable to keep up the struggle to be active, and others who were not prepared to do it. The result was that many residents did not live up to expectations, expectations that they believed in as well as staff.

Mr Jepson is an example of someone caught in this conflict. At interview he talked about keeping going and doing things for himself. Occasionally he turned down offers of help because he felt he had to do things for himself. Frequently he despaired of what he had become in his own eyes, as well as everyone else's: 'to come to this'.

The hypothesis that emerges from this follows from Gubrium's socio-environmental theory of ageing (see p. 7 above). Residents will be satisfied with their life-style when their resources are sufficient to meet the norms of their immediate community. Thus it could be that everybody accepted that it was important to keep active in old age and the individual resident had the physical and the material resources to accomplish this. Alternatively a resident may choose a more contemplative life-style, 'a rocking-chair type' existence (Havighurst, 1968). This also will lead to satisfaction provided others agree that this is reasonable.

A problem emerges when the expectations of staff, the expectations of residents, or the performance of residents do not match. In Mr Jepson's case his performance could not match the expectations of himself and those around him, including other residents. There are similarities to the analysis provided by Miller and Gwynne (1972) who discuss different models of caring for the physically handicapped. Their conclusion is that the most appropriate model is an organisational model in which staff support the resident in her chosen way of life. Thus a resident may choose independence or dependence and will be supported by staff in the choice she has made.

The parallel situation in an old people's home would be that a resident might choose activity or disengagement and would be supported in that choice by staff. The task of the residential worker becomes that of enabling others to live in the way they wish.

It is at this point that the stop-go economy provides a useful analogy. Staff get satisfaction from looking after highly dependent people. The new resident arrives at the home *having already adjusted her picture of herself*, seeing herself as 'the type of person who has to live in a home'. The staff enjoy looking after the new resident and, for this reason and that of organisational convenience, make decisions for the resident and carry out tasks for her. The resident adds to her own anticipation of the home the myriad of subtle messages that inform her of what is expected of her. The range of expectations leads to her doing very little for herself – whether it is clearing a table, making her bed, or even making decisions.

The consequence of this range of factors – the uneasy role of the very old in our society, the giving up prior to admission, the needs and wishes of staff and the decreasing physical ability of the resident – is the very picture of the old age home quoted earlier: 'armchairs in rooms around the edge of the wall, just sitting. The sad thing about the whole thing is that patients sit there from choice.'

In the preceding paragraphs I have been trying to illustrate a pattern and have not been making a general statement about all residents and all staff at The Pines. However, the pattern is important. Residents live in a situation where they do little. Others, those who have helped to create the situation, whether as staff, relatives, or other professionals, are uneasy at the picture. They attempt to stimulate the resident into activity. Mrs Draxton did very little. 'We need to keep going as much as possible, but there is nothing to keep us going' she said to me in an interview. Staff endeavoured to motivate her to some activity, achieved little success, gave up and dismissed her as the misery she knows she is.

The stop-go regime is neither successful nor satisfying in either stage. In particular the attempts to reactivate after the resident has been encouraged to stop are emotionally exhausting and doomed to failure. The discrepancy is further highlighted by the contrast between the staff statements about those things that it would be good for the residents to do (see pp. 153–4 above) and the little amount actually done by the residents.

Fundamentally there is uncertainty about what people ought to do and it must be remembered that the institution will receive some of those who have found the process of ageing hardest of all. The uncertainty that exists in the wider society about ageing has already been mentioned but must be recalled here. More people are living longer; there is less need for them to work and less work available either within families or in occupations; without a clear role the old have to make a major readjustment of their life-style and picture of self; there is uncertainty as to which pattern or patterns of adjustment are most satisfactory.

This uncertainty exists in relation to the old, those over retirement age. If, however, we consider the very old the uncertainties are even greater. Worsening health becomes more significant after 75 and the prospect of the weariness and struggle that make up the daily living of some very old people is daunting. So it is hard to consider successful ageing in such a context.

We need to face the reality of this situation. The institution cannot solve many of these problems. Miss Brinton talked about her memories of the First World War. Her fiancée had been killed and she had never married. The memory, sixty years later, was still powerful but even more so was the bitterness as she stated that she would not need to be in a home if only she had married and had children. The home cannot solve that, any more than it can solve the crippling arthritis of another resident.

Within the home as good and as appropriate a life-style as is possible can be offered, but the home should not be under pressure to *solve* everything. Similarly it is necessary for staff not to offer the same way of managing the situation to all residents. Therefore staff must not look for one pattern of successful ageing within the home, particularly because such a pattern would be likely to reflect their own perception of how they would cope.

STYLES OF AGEING

Havighurst (1968) suggests eight patterns of ageing. They are all deduced from a study within the wider community but are a useful starting point for considering styles of ageing within the institution. Its eight groups were:

Reorganisers	They reorganise their lives to substitute new activities for lost ones
Focused	They are well integrated, with medium levels of activity, and select one or two role areas.
Successful disengaged	They have low activity levels with high satisfaction. A contented 'rocking-chair' position.
Holding on	They hold on as long as possible to the activities of middle age, and have high satisfaction as long as this works.
Constricted	They have reduced their role activity but are less-integrated personalities than the *focused* group.
Succourance-seeking	They are successful in getting emotional support from others and thus maintain a medium level of role activity and of life satisfaction.
Apathetic	They have low role activity combined with medium or low life satisfaction. Presumably they are people who have never given much to life and never expected much.
Disorganised	They have deteriorated thought processes and poor control over their emotions. They barely maintain themselves in the community and have low or, at the most, medium life satisfaction.

Havighurst examined three dimensions – activity, life satisfaction and personality – and concluded that personality was 'the pivotal dimension in describing patterns of ageing and in predicting relationships between level of activity and life satisfaction'.

It must be remembered that he appears to assume that inability to survive in the community is itself a sign of low satisfaction. However, his approach of considering how people relate their present life-style to that of the past is useful. In relating this to the old age institution we can consider the way an individual's life-style within the home relates to her past pattern of life.

The first dimension to consider is the extent to which links are maintained with family and community. It has been argued that links with family drop off once an individual arrives in a residential home. In this study I did not examine differences in family involvement but was surprised at the extent of continuing visiting. Many relatives visited several times a week, some every day. Of course nothing can replace the continual contact when living with relatives but I would suspect that most other people were visited at least as often by close relatives as they had been before. This is not to say that residents did not wish for more visits. Mrs Draxton would sit wondering why her daughter had not visited, but that pattern would have been as likely to exist had she been living with anybody else.

By contrast, links with neighbours, friends, or groups of people (churches and clubs) were far more tenuous. In this area styles of ageing are significant. Mrs Williams's powerful statement about role reversal – 'You see, I used to come to sing to the people here' – explains why she found it hard to receive visitors from church, though she did maintain some contacts. Mrs Smith took the initiative in cutting off links with past groups. It may be argued that deliberately cutting off contact with others from the community is a defence against possible rejection by them. However, it is clear that the predominant reason stated by the residents was that they did not wish to be seen as a resident of an old age home.

So some people chose to cut off links with the community and a few wanted to cut off links with their own past. 'I didn't want a lot of my old things around me' said Mrs Pinker. 'I preferred to start with new.'

The second dimension to consider is activity within the home. Some residents would help others; some would carry out tasks for themselves (e.g. making beds); some would carry out work for the group (e.g. drying up). But the pattern of activity for the individual is also important. 'Activity' is a broad term but could be considered in a more thorough way than was undertaken in this study. Some factors to consider would be the following:

Amount of movement Moving around within the home, short walks around the building, walking to the town.
Range of activities The number of different activities undertaken by an individual – including personal tasks for self (washing, etc.), tasks for others, hobbies (reading, knitting, watching TV), involvement with groups within the home on a formal or informal basis, and similarly with outside groups, contact with family and friends.
Investment in particular activities The importance attached to the activity by the resident.

A third category to examine is that of personality type. Here again Havighurst's work is valuable. He considers both the cognitive and affective aspects of personality and emerges with four major types – integrated, armoured-defended, passive-dependent, unintegrated. (The eight patterns already mentioned are developments from these four groupings.)

Finally the life satisfaction of the individual can be tested to record

the extent to which a person (*a*) finds satisfaction in the activities of his everyday life; (b) regards his life as meaningful and accepts both the good and the bad in it; (c) feels that he has succeeded in achieving his major goals; (d) has a positive image of himself; and (e) maintains happy and optimistic moods and attitudes. (Havighurst, 1968)

The life satisfaction test used in this study emerged from his work.

How far are Havighurst's personality patterns useful in considering old people in institutions? They are a valuable starting point but some provisos need to be built in. At The Pines there were some people with medium to high levels of activity (within the context of the organisation) who had low levels of satisfaction – they endeavoured to keep going but the activities had insufficient meaning for them. Mrs Smith and Mrs Roberts both fell into this category. The latter is a particularly important example because she was not as bitter as Mrs Smith about life, in fact found plenty of situations which she enjoyed, but was basically dissatisfied with her life in relation to the past: 'It's a pity you have to get old. Why do you have to suffer? I have got all these aches and pains.' She stated that the most important thing in her life was to get rid of her aches and pains and that past times were happier.

Mrs Williams illustrates a different situation. She kept active but did not invest the activities with a lot of meaning. 'It fills in time' was one of her frequent comments about her knitting, but she thought that her continual knitting of tea-cosies was rather futile.

Secondly, Havighurst's concentration on personality does not allow for the cumulative effect of calamities. Tobin and Lieberman (1976) give examples of situations where the accumulation of events seemed to over-ride personality. Certainly at The Pines great difficulty in moving around was associated with low levels of satisfaction. The correlation was not invariable but there was a tendency for the weariness to be carried over to low satisfaction.

Thirdly, there is need for a category who are *detached*. These people may not be apathetic and are further removed from involvement than the 'successful disengaged'. At one end of the spectrum they might be regarded as *having given up* or *having despaired*, at the other they have accepted their withdrawal and are really *ready for death*.

In addition there is certainly need for a category who have been *holders-on* but have failed to hold on. They are not so much apathetic as *disillusioned*.

The prominence of passivity in Havighurst's analysis is interesting, for Tobin and Lieberman find this the most significant factor in death or poor adjustment on entry to a residential home. They point out that 'because the rewarded style is assertiveness, additional stress is placed on passive residents to change their typical adaptational pattern'. At The Pines those who were most active and assertive were regarded by staff as the best models of ageing; in addition those who were determined in their behaviour, for example, about not leaving their bedrooms, succeeded in getting their own way.

It is here that a discrepancy is illustrated again. Staff rated highly those residents who kept going and did things for themselves; yet they got satisfaction from helping the dependent. In fact they probably had two pictures of a model resident – the first would be the person who kept active; the second would be someone who was highly dependent but uncomplaining.

At The Pines the average life satisfaction score was 13. The test successfully discriminated between residents with Mr Jepson scoring only 7 and Mrs Pinker as the most satisfied with 20. Since I know the results of no other use of the test in residential homes it is not possible to make comparisons.

However, Peace *et al.* (1979), using different scales (indices of affect balance and of satisfaction with home life), do consider factors which explain satisfaction. They point out that satisfaction with home life was not linked to the degree of choice held by the resident and that it was those residents who conformed most to expected standards who were most satisfied. This would tie in with Gubrium's analysis in which people were said to have high morale when resources and norms matched.

OLD AGE AND ITS MEANING TO DIFFERENT PEOPLE

Sometimes staff tried to get unwilling people to do things, such as puzzles, or to join in activities. These illustrate the tension between caring and coercing and the uncertainty about one's right to intervene.

Residents responded to ageing in different ways. There were few who fitted neatly into categories: Mrs Richardson, stating that people at The Pines should not be worried by their relatives' concerns and that she was happy to keep going as long as possible but then glad to give up, is the only example of the successful disengaged. Miss Carpenter, who revelled in all the bustle and activities, was the only person who could be classified as a reorganiser.

Most others felt more strongly either rejection, by family or society, or the burden of old age. They adapted to this in different ways but entering an institution did mean having to present oneself in a new situation. In fact at times the whole of life seemed to be a presentation, with conscious planning of one's reactions to different events. For some the important thing was not to display their feelings of sadness; for others it was to keep at bay their feelings of purposelessness, feelings that might be compounded by the few demands made on them. Some were clear that it was difficult to adjust to their changed ability: 'The difference isn't the home, it's me.' Mr Jepson said that he couldn't understand what had happened to part of his brain.

For these old people, maybe because their lives had been harsher than those of the population at large, maybe because they saw infirmity all around them, questions about purpose and suffering were common. 'Why should it happen to me?'; 'I must have been very bad for this to happen' were examples of the questioning of religion which takes place at times of tragedy. Some had few supports in other parts of their lives to help them make sense of things.

There were a group also for whom their belief in God was the solid aspect of their lives, which put their pain or suffering into perspective. Some stated that life was wearisome and that they would be happy to die.

The focus here has been on *ageing* in an institution rather than on the effects of the institution. In this respect it is important to re-emphasise the relief of residents at being looked after. Nearly all were glad for the physical care of themselves, the provision of meals and the warmth.

One response to the uncertainties about the process of ageing was to venerate age itself. 'She's a wonderful age' or 'she's wonderful for her age', were examples of this. The personality or the quality of the action were ignored – the focus became age which allowed some of the tensions to be ignored. When Mrs White died at 89 her son's response was 'I was sorry she didn't make ninety'.

Another aspect of ageing of great significance in the institution is the need to communicate about bodily functioning. The language used to discuss this was that remembered from childhood, 'I want to do a wee', 'I've done my job' said Mr Jepson. The real problem is to find a language that is appropriate and that does not lead to infantilising.

In fact one of the key tasks in old age homes is to provide for the physical needs of dependent people, whether helping to wash, eat, walk, or go to the lavatory, *without* reducing the status of the old to that of children. The temptation is to assume, as did some of the staff at The Pines, that 'they're like children really'. This leads to patronising, to a belief that their concerns are trivial, to authoritarianism and inappropriate control.

An earlier section demonstrated the control at The Pines of social contact between men and women. Important in this is the smaller number of men in residential homes. However, it is apparent that living in a residential home offers for those with few contacts more opportunities for close contact with others, especially others of the opposite sex, than would have existed prior to admission. Alongside this must be placed our increased knowledge about sexuality in later life (see Puner, 1974; Felstein, 1973; Hendricks and Hendricks, 1977). All these sources make it clear that sexual intercourse is more common among the old than had previously been thought. It is argued that psychological aspects are far more important than physical changes in people's attitudes to sex for the elderly.

The subject is important because of the assumptions made by others about the old. Puner outlines the cruel caricatures that are held about 'dirty old men' and 'old maids'. In the residential institution the attitudes of staff have immense significance. That is not to say that men and women in an old age home *will* want to develop sexual relationships with others – simply that they *may*, and that staff should know that this is not abnormal and face squarely any uncertainties they may have as to what is acceptable. At The Pines the possibility of such a relationship was discouraged in its early stages.

The final aspect to be examined here concerns *assumptions* about ageing. Most people considered greater activity would lead to increased satisfaction. 'No wonder that group of men are miserable', said a local doctor, 'there's so much inactivity.' The converse of this was the assumption that those who were active were the most satisfied. This was not always accurate and therefore staff need to consider the validity of their bases for assessment. The assumption of some members of staff that one confused resident, Mrs Hendon, was happy because she did not know what was going on was similarly inaccurate. In fact the interview showed that she was completely in touch with her feelings of unhappiness about living in a home.

Assumptions are made also about appropriate behaviour. Words like 'depression' are used too readily and this leads to poor diagnosis, especially when coupled with assertions such as 'depression is only to be expected in old age'. On the other hand it is necessary to be aware that neither medicine nor social work can take away all the feelings of sadness or wearisomeness. Yet that knowledge does not excuse the doctor who talked to Mrs Black about how she felt. 'How old are you?' he asked. 'Ninety-three' she replied. 'You don't need a doctor; you need a magician' he retorted.

Chapter 12

THE FUNCTION OF OLD AGE HOMES

THE PINES AND THE TYPOLOGY

It was soon apparent that The Pines did not fit neatly into any cell of the grid formed from the two variables: (1) attitude to ageing, (2) degree of control of life-style.

Staff believed that people are happiest when they have plenty to do. Visitors were despondent at the sight of residents sitting and doing little. Residents felt that they should be doing more. Yet attempts to stimulate activity often failed – residents might not want to join in the singing, to go on an outing, to exercise their legs, or to do a puzzle. The reason lies partly in the way residents had altered their self-picture before admission to an extent that was difficult to change. Residents were deprived of roles they thought to be valid (parent, spouse, worker, community member) and many could find nothing to do which they believed to be worthwhile. Activity for its own sake, knitting tea-cosies that nobody wants, is worthless.

Similarly, disengaging because one cannot find anything worthwhile in which to engage is not likely to lead to happiness. So residents who sat back and had things done for them were not more content.

The third model of ageing, the socio-environmental, examines the extent to which resources and expectations match. However, it is possible to have the resources to meet the expectations of *others* but remain dissatisfied with one's life. Mrs Roberts, who organised the football pontoon and went out to the pub, was thought by staff to manage her life successfully, but *she* thought her life fairly pointless.

A conversation I had with Mrs Loosely illustrates the way in which an over-riding tension, in this case brought about by her wish to be back in her own home, prohibits any style of ageing being successful. She told me that she was depressed because of worrying about her own home; she had locked up but not done any shopping (it was now about *eight months* after her admission, but it needs to be remembered that she wished to go home and was manipulated by all parties into staying). She repeated at least ten times that she would ask the doctor and see if he would agree to her going home. He had said 'Get someone in', and she had got a young couple to live in the house but they had not bothered to call in to see her. She would like someone to live with her but it was difficult to get people.

'You can be happy here but it's so lonely. People don't drop in so much, there's nothing to do.' She saw one of the staff come by with a pile of rags. 'That's the sort of thing I like doing, cleaning up cupboards. If I stay in here long enough, I'll never walk. I could walk down to the shops at home.'

ME: (knowing that staff encouraged her to walk) You could walk here.
MRS L: Yes but it's not the same, I don't like going out on my own.

She talked about her past charity work, how she had collected for various charities including the old workhouse. She had given a lot of money for a prize for a whist drive once – 'I used to like playing cards' she went on.

ME: Would you like to play now? I could find a pack.
MRS L: No I don't think so, I don't feel like it.

I suggested pushing her out in her wheelchair to look round the town, which I had done several times, but she didn't want that.

ME: Couldn't you bring a few things from your own home here?
MRS L: No, I don't want to muddle them up.

She continued by discussing the TV programmes which she watched, though the doctor had said she shouldn't because it was bad for her eyes. Knowing that she had plenty of money I suggested she might get a radio. No, she wouldn't do that, though she would like to listen if she had one.

The GP was insistent that she could not manage at home. Nobody was prepared to instigate formal legal proceedings under the National Assistance Act to compel her to stay and nobody was prepared to tell her that she had the right to go home whenever she wished. The message of my conversation with her that day was quite clear, though it seemed to take me a long time to grasp – until the basic tension was resolved she had little enthusiasm for anything else.

Any general picture of The Pines must push the differences of individuals beneath the surface. Mrs Pinker kept active and was happy; Miss Carpenter loved all the activities; Mrs Richardson was pleased to put up her feet and have a rest. Each of these individuals had achieved ego-integration (Erikson) or a resolution of their present state in terms of their whole life. Such resolution may be realised through activity or disengagement, but without such resolution both activity and disengagement will be sterile.

At The Pines, staff, residents and outsiders predominantly believed in keeping active, in finding things to do. However, only a few believed that there were worthwhile tasks for the very old to perform. Most thought activity was better than inactivity. It must be remembered that the actions of staff did not always endorse their statements. The staff were prepared to do so much for residents that there was little residents needed to do for themselves. There were also some staff who thought that to be mildly confused, like Mrs Hendon, arguably an extreme form of disengagement, was a good way to grow old, though Mrs Hendon's own comments suggested she was not as happy as staff thought.

The second variable, control of life-style, showed a wider spread. The *minimum control by residents* was evident in staff entering rooms without knocking and putting away clothes that had been left around, holding centrally of drugs and pension books, staff deciding who sits where at meal-times and in sitting areas, and planning the decor of rooms.

Medium level of control by residents was far more the pattern – there were few strict rules, though norms were influential; residents did not hold their pension books but could spend their money how they liked; there were no bath rotas and residents had some ability to negotiate bath-times; residents could choose their own doctors but staff were intermediaries in deciding whether a doctor should be called; they could carpet their rooms but had to leave the carpet behind; they had little formal influence over menus (though staff would notice what was popular) but they were free to eat what they wished (again with some provisos); they could use their own bedrooms at most times of the day; they could choose which clothes to wear, though there was an expectation that the men would wear ties.

Maximum control of life-style by the resident was shown by freedom for visitors to call at any time, freedom for residents to plan their own day (with some provisos, particularly that the more passive would be encouraged to join in certain events), freedom for residents to go out when they wished.

The Pines fitted mostly into the 'activity' column of the grid, with the dominant cell being that of the therapeutic unit, while the nursing home and retirement community had equal influence. At the same time the preparedness to do things for residents and the occasional acknowledgement that residents responded to ageing differently show the influence of disengagement and socio-environmental theories. Figure 12.1 shows how The Pines spreads across several cells rather than fits neatly into any one.

Figure 12.1 *Typology of homes*

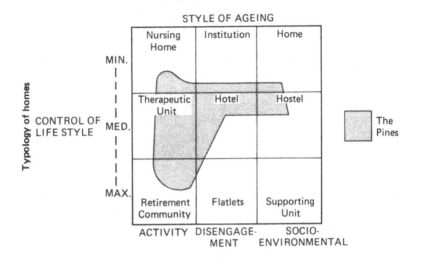

LIMITATIONS OF THIS TYPOLOGY

Thus the grid provides a useful framework for examining the practice of an institution. The details of the original typology (pp. 22–7 above) added some description to each cell. Consequently in each cell there were details derived from the variables about ageing and control of life-style but also statements about staffing (e.g. hierarchy and types of training) and the philosophy of the unit. While neat pictures of model units were produced, too many variables were created to be acceptable for a two-dimensional grid. The Pines, for example, had an activity model of ageing with a medium level of control by residents as its dominant mode. Thus it fitted most easily into the cell named the therapeutic unit. However, The Pines did not have a belief in treatment and rehabilitation, nor did it have a head of home who was social work trained, two factors which I had ascribed to the therapeutic unit. The grid could be used more precisely if it had been limited to information which could be derived from the variables.

However important these two variables are, there are also other aspects which need consideration. Tobin and Lieberman (1976) asked a group of people waiting for admission to old age homes which factors they thought important in contemplating admission. Eighty-three per cent included *care* in their reply, 66 per cent mentioned *activity*, 60 per cent spoke of *people*, 43 per cent referred to *privacy* and 30 per cent picked out *freedom*.

Residents at The Pines also stressed *care* as a central concern. Under this heading they were glad to have people to do things for them such as bathing or helping them to get to bed, and also glad to have staff around. Taking this into account, measures of the quality and consistency of the care provided would be useful analytic tools, for residents have a right to reliable care. For example, flexibility of arrangements for bathing, a valid objective, must not lead to an inconsistency of service. Indeed, flexibility should lead to discriminating between residents in the way the service is provided. But a particular resident might choose an unvarying pattern of service. In spite of limits as to flexibility, The Pines would have rated highly in the quality and consistency of care.

ANALYSIS OF OBJECTIVES

Several staff stated the aim of the home should be the happiness of residents: 'a happy home', 'happy and contented residents' were two such answers. Individuality was also mentioned: 'making residents feel each is an individual, their happiness and well-being the most important objective'. Another's response was 'to help the residents live a normal and independent life', similar to the local authority's goal, 'the maintenance and promotion of the independence of the individual'. Other aims were 'making good links with the community', 'providing a welcome for visitors', 'enriching lives as much as possible' and 'helping to die with dignity and peacefully'. Significantly residents also predominantly thought of the purpose of the establishment as 'making people happy' and 'providing a home'.

Much of the physical care was good. Since that is one of the most important needs of residents, then meeting this adequately will enhance the likelihood of residents' happiness. And it should be noted that there was concern for people in the way the provision was made. However, there are strong counter-arguments to an assumption that provision of services is all that matters. Many residents scored low in the life satisfaction tests or talked about their frustrations and unhappiness. In addition the way the care was provided might lead to dependence rather than the stated aim of independence.

There was a tendency for organisational goals, those concerned with 'the machinery by which the society continues to operate', to predominate over both instrumental goals, those aiming at skill development, and expressive goals, concerned with moral or religious states or an individual's need for esteem and acceptance (Millham et al., 1975b).

Thus senior staff gave a lot of time to ensuring that the place was clean and tidy – hence the morning inspection round by senior staff and the time taken over ordering and distributing stores. Menu-planning, producing staffing rotas and other administrative tasks also took up considerable senior staff time. Care attendants commented that they would have liked more staff available at times of peak demand but there was a suggestion that the rota met their needs to get overtime. Timing of events was important – meals were never late and on one occasion when the tea was put back a quarter of an hour so that a television programme might be watched it caused concern amongst staff rather than residents.

Visitors were discouraged from the physical care of the residents because it upset the staffing system: a clear example of a situation where the need to arrange the task to suit staff conflicted with the care of the residents. Similarly staff often informally discouraged residents from the independence the home was supposed to promote. Meal-times, with staff having to clear tables rapidly, are another example of this.

Coffee mornings were held two or three times a year – the residents made little for the stalls, did not run them and few went to the event because it was so crowded. Staff did most of the work, helped by the Friends both beforehand and on the day. It appeared a way of making money (its main aim) and of building the reputation of the establishment.

THE FUNCTION OF THE OLD AGE HOME

The information given in Chapter 5 suggested that there were two main patterns that led to admission. (1) People who lived alone became unable to manage daily living tasks (climbing stairs, cooking, washing), mostly because of their own physical incapacity but also because of mental confusion or bad housing. The situation of Mrs Loosely illustrates this – according to reports she found it difficult to get around, was forgetful, failed to look after herself properly; in addition her house was not very suitable. (2) Where people lived with others (usually family, in particular children) the situation of either old person or 'caregiver' changed, often following a spell in hospital.

Given these pictures, what needs must be met? The first is for suitable housing for the frail old; the second is for support in the tasks of daily living; the third is for oversight, which in the case of Mrs Loosely may mean constant attendance and with others may be less frequent.

The temptation is to try to meet these needs through major shifts of social policy, an approach adopted by Townsend (1962) and Meacher (1972), who envisage the abolition of residential homes. This appears an unlikely answer because residents of homes are more frail than previously (dramatically different since Townsend's survey), because of the increase in numbers of frail elderly, likely to continue to the end of this century, and, more prosaically, because we have the establishments, and people will want to use them.

Certainly the number of residents of old age homes who could manage in minimum-support schemes, such as sheltered bungalows with wardens on call or similar housing association schemes, is small. The majority need a substantial number of services.

Consequently the prime function of the home should be *to provide a living base in which basic physical needs are met in a way which allows the individual the maximum potential for achieving mastery*. This definition starts from the need for suitable housing and the need for support in the tasks of daily living. Since this is the expressed need of the client it is worth repeating that this must be the starting point for discovering the objectives of residential homes.

Alongside this, however, it is essential to remember that too often the provision of such support services has lessened the independence and destroyed the individuality of the recipient. The examples in earlier chapters demonstrate this. The statement must be taken in its entirety – it is *not* saying that the function of the home is only to provide for physical needs. The essential task is to provide such services in a way that *offers the opportunity* for an individual to be in command of her own life – and it must be noted that the individual is not to be forced to assume such command.

Since such a statement of function may call forth strong reaction it is legitimate to examine further the rationale that lies behind it. The statement is derived from the reasons given by residents for their need for admission. Much of its firmness derives from this seemingly simple comment. Barbara Wootton (1959) attacked social workers for presuming that they knew better than their clients what were their real needs. A similar temptation exists for residential workers with the elderly and the temptation is magnified when they look to field social work or residential social work with children for clarification of their task. Treatment, change and development are key words that are likely to arise from those disciplines. They are not the central task of residential work with the elderly.

The client who enters an old age home has *not* done so because she wishes to be helped with the resolution of intrapersonal or interpersonal problems. In this way residential homes can be seen to be on a continuum that starts with living in one's own home, has a middle stage of sheltered housing, followed by residential homes and perhaps hospitalisation at the end. Residential homes, then, should be seen as housing, with services provided.

Another value of the definition above is that it allows escape from the assumption that an old age home should meet all the needs of the elderly. Such assumptions start from considering old age, proceed to draw up a list of the needs of the elderly and then plan ways of running a home to meet such needs. This seems caring and humanitarian. Yet it is didactic and authoritarian. If residential work is based on such assumptions we end up treating those who have no wish to be treated, attempting to change someone who has not understood that to be the reason why she has gone into a home.

The definition stated earlier is concerned with the *focus* of the task; it is not commenting on the complexity or simplicity of the task. In fact to provide a living base and services in a way that maximises someone's independence is both complex and skilled.

In considering that task we must recognise some of the pros and cons of residential living as expressed by residents and workers. The pros included: the comfort and warmth; being glad to have a break; having things like washing and ironing done for you; having nothing to worry about; the security, especially of having staff available; the satisfaction of having something to eat; companionship and something going on. The last two items were mentioned more by outsiders than residents. The anxieties were: lack of privacy; fear of regimentation; the loss of one's independence; having to live with other people; and being without one's familiar possessions. Residents mentioned fewer of these items at interview but my observation suggested that they were all of concern to residents.

Before looking in detail at the implications of this definition it is worth making some general points. Though happiness may be a legitimate goal for individual old people, as Margaret Tilley (1971) suggests, it is not sufficient as the goal for an old people's home. Miller and Gwynne (1972) wrote about homes for the handicapped that they

were not satisfied by notions of 'happiness', which for us could have connotations of passivity. The subjective comparisons we found ourselves making when we visited institutions had more to do with a quality of 'aliveness'. In some establishments, inmates were probing their environment, questioning assumptions, using their capacities. In many others, the inmates seemed to be inhabiting a shrunken world; the majority were moribund.

While sharing their enthusiasm for a home in which such 'aliveness' exists, I do not consider it should be the central task of an old age establishment. The old are entitled to be 'detached' or disengaged. Their earlier statement – that it is 'the task of the institution, without either destroying the inmate's individuality or denying his dependence, to provide a setting in which he can find his own best way of relating to the external world and to himself' – is more satisfactory.

An intention behind my definition, which would be implicit in Miller and Gwynne's above, is to make it clear to staff that they do not have full responsibility for assessing and planning an individual's life. Consequently, and crucially, they do not carry the full burden of those who are unhappy. Some people will continue to be bitter in a well-run establishment although I believe that 'happiness' and 'aliveness' will be by-products for most residents of such an organisation.

Another premise to my definition is that high quality of the service is essential. Therefore, if we take the example of bathing, the bathing is to be of a high standard (staff must know how to lift and make someone feel secure) and must create the opportunity for the individual to assert mastery. To repeat – the task in terms of my definition is both complex and skilful.

The components of the task are: (1) the provision of a living base; (2) the meeting of basic physical needs; (3) the enhancement of a potential for mastery. These components will be considered separately though there is some interaction between them as, for example, when poor planning of a bathroom makes it difficult for a resident to bath herself.

(1)   *The provision of a living base*

For most people the residential home needs to be seen as their home for the rest of their life. While it may be encouraging to hope for rehabilitation and return to other living situations, in reality few residents are able or willing to move away. Comparisons with ordinary housing situations are useful (Clough, 1979a and b). The person who buys a new house keeps possession for as long as she wishes; someone renting will still have substantial rights as tenant, and cannot be moved at the whim of the landlord. It is the security of tenure of the tenant that the resident needs. At this point it is useful to reflect on the terminology used. I am arguing for the use of terms similar to those in normal situations – hence 'house' and 'tenant' – as a way of reducing both stigma and dependency, a point made by Whittaker (1979) in relation to residential child care. But such terms are also valuable because they encourage us to expect the same rights for a resident as for any other tenant, unless good reason can be shown to the contrary. Therefore the resident should be able to treat her room as her own, able to decorate it, to have a key to it, to use it when she wishes for herself or to entertain her friends. It is *her* room. Even those who share a room may use it more if they feel it is their room.

It is sometimes forgotten that one's home is the place for relaxation and informality as well as moments that are more clearly private or intimate. Events such as reading the paper, putting one's feet up, dozing in a chair, knitting, watching the television, chatting with friends, are typically carried out in the intimacy of home, even though they may not be specifically private. Within a residential home they are typically carried out in the semi-public lounge, so it is not surprising that they are unlikely to lead to close contact between people.

The bed-sitting rooms should become the private base for residents, in spite of the pitifully small size of bedrooms in most modern homes.

Even in these, placing the bed against a wall may make a room more usable as a bed-sitting room, though of course a resident who needs assistance from two staff to get in or out of bed will need the bed in a central position. Using one's room more as a private base means that the individual has less fear of an invasion of privacy and a greater opportunity to avoid other people.

In terms of future planning it is necessary to build larger single bed-sitting rooms, even at the cost of fewer or smaller group sitting rooms. (Lipman and Slater, 1977, illustrate the influence planning may have on style of living.)

(2) *The meeting of basic physical needs*

Residents at The Pines considered this the main reason for their admission. It involves ensuring that various needs are met – staff may need to carry out some jobs completely, help residents to complete others. leave residents alone in other situations.

It is to be noted also how glad some residents were not to have to look after the fabric of a building, to be free from worry about both bills and heating, how pleased they were to have a rest or break, to be warm and comfortable.

The processes with which residents may need help are: getting up and going to bed, dressing, bathing and washing, going to the lavatory, washing clothes, ironing, mending, cleaning, bed-making, provision of drinks, snacks and main meals, laying tables and washing up, emptying commodes, assistance with walking or getting into a wheel-chair.

Meals provide an example where there is a rich variety of possibilities, although there will be constraints in forms of building and facilities, money and people. Starting with the wishes of the resident – a resident may wish to cook all meals herself, to cook some meals herself, to cook no meals herself. She may wish for help in preparing some meals. She may want meals at a range of different times and may choose to go without some meals. She may wish to eat the meal in the privacy of her own room, with a friend, or a group in the dining hall. This is not the recipe for chaos it may sound. First, relatives or friends may be prepared to help, may even bring in meals; secondly, staff might have to do less cooking and less supervision of meals; thirdly, we must acknowledge that there will be constraints on what is possible. My contention is that we should start from the choice and then examine what is possible, so that the planning takes account of what is wanted, not the way staff think the task is best carried out for residents or themselves.

It is apparent that routines may at times be counter-productive in terms of staff time. For example, frail residents at The Pines were got up early (remember the senior staff member saying 'Poor Mrs Tinley sat in the lounge at seven a.m., sleeping in her chair, it's such a long day for her'), helped in to breakfast and at 10 o'clock might be taken back to the bathroom and undressed for a bath. Getting up later, a light breakfast in bed and then a bath would be kinder and simpler. In addition several residents would have liked to stay in bed for longer and not had breakfast. Pressure on staff would have been eased.

Other needs discussed in Chapter 6 were: money, medicine, doctors, the daily programme. The premise here should be that these are the concern of the resident. The resident may request help from friend, relative, or staff, and there may need to be some negotiations as to what help can be offered. Incidentally the money must be referred to as *pension*, not pocket money. As far as is possible residents should be treated as if in their own homes. Thus if a doctor considers a particular resident unable to manage her own medicines, even with a special dispenser, then he will need to find someone to look after them for her.

In situations where a resident is being helped or having a service provided the resident is dependent on staff for the manner in which the service is performed. One danger is that staff may meet physical needs in a way that creates dependence, and this must be avoided whenever possible.

Residents frequently mentioned how pleased they were to have people around if something went wrong. The tension created by worrying about what might happen can itself be a cause of accidents, so another task for the unit is to ensure that staff are available and that there is an alarm system, should people fall.

One of the fears people have of residential living is of regimentation. Therefore residents should be regimented as little as possible when being cared for. Resulting from less regimentation would be a reduction in the occasions when large groups of residents are assembled together. The frailties of old age would be less conspicuous.

In areas concerned with dependence, security and regimentation this section merges with the next. Physical and psycho-social needs interact.

(3) *The enhancement of a potential for mastery*
The very existence of the old age home can be a factor in enhancing mastery. People may be able to do more for themselves because the facilities are more suitable than in their own homes; there will be more time for other things if the resident does not have to work at all the tasks of daily living; it is possible to take more risks if a person knows that there are staff available to help. The home itself provides potential for mastery, as well as a potential for dependence.

One fact that was apparent from this study was the way in which residents struggled to maintain integrity and status. Residents often adopted one of two patterns of response. In the first the resident asserted her dissimilarity from other residents – that she was younger, healthier, or less confused. To make the point clear she might criticise the behaviour of other residents. The second approach is to demonstrate one's worth in terms of outside contacts – the people one used to know, the number of visitors one has. Hopefully a greater control of one's life would lead to a reduction in the need to resort to such damaging mechanisms.

Similarly I have argued that residents may be defeated before arrival at a home. Prospective residents need support if they are not to alter their perceptions of themselves and their life-style before they enter the residential home. At present many people enter residential homes believing that they must adapt to the way the home runs. And while there is some truth in that – any change demands adaptation – it is also apparent that a greater variety of life-style is possible. Staff in homes comment that they know very little about a resident's past life. Even a good report from the field social worker has only brief comments on the ways in which someone actually lived and many reports are poor. In any case, better reporting serves only to provide the staff with better information and leaves to the staff the task of attempting to motivate.

There is a need to help prospective residents consider their present life-style (i.e. before admission) and to plan for their life within the home. Elsewhere (Clough, 1978d) I have discussed ways of building up a picture of someone's way of living. This would pick up treasured moments – a hot water bottle at night-time, listening to *Woman's Hour* after lunch – and difficult moments. It would illustrate the way daily living tasks are tackled and include activities and interests. Some themes might emerge, for example, how someone manages loneliness or handicap, and some important events that happen less frequently.

Having this information, it becomes possible to think with the resident about how she would wish to live when she moves to the residential home. 'Which parts of her life would she wish to hang on to if possible? Which parts would she change?' would be two key questions. Thus the prospective resident is thinking about the detail of her life so that she may continue to manage her life in the way she wishes.

However good the planning, the resident will need support at the time of entering a residential home. Bowlby (1951), followed by Robertson, illustrated the patterns of adaptation made by children when admitted to a residential unit. The significance of their work was in showing that the quiet child, one who had been through stages of despair, anger and denial and had become apathetic, was regarded by many staff as having made a successful adjustment to the home or hospital ward. The clear implication, endorsed by more recent writing on crisis intervention, is that it is necessary to work with the resident *during the crisis of admission* (moving home is a life-crisis for many other people) and not to wait until she has settled down.

A secondary issue concerns the status of the person who helps to compile the 'map' or plan. This might be the old person, the residential or field worker, a relative, or a friend. Whichever person is involved, it is necessary to consider what should be shared with staff. The essential point is that applicants need to be as fully involved in the decision to be admitted as possible (those who said they had made the decision themselves were the more satisfied at The Pines). Once the decision has been made, residents-to-be must be involved in planning for the future and for the type of life they wish to lead. They need to consider the resources available to maintain links between themselves and friends, clubs or churches, since once the break has been made it is much harder to make new links and people may give up and not make the effort. More time should be allowed for people to reach decisions and plan their next stage than is sometimes given.

One of the central findings of this study is the influence on practice of one's own attitude to ageing. The residential workers and outside professionals overwhelmingly favoured the activity model of ageing (finding work like activities to replace those one gives up). This influenced their attitude to residents and, coupled with the residential workers' own wishes to care for the dependent, made for considerable confusion. Other evidence points to the fact that there is no single successful model of ageing. Therefore the task for staff is to encourage the individual to decide how she wants to live.

The right of the resident to be treated as she wishes was the theme of a short article by Clough and Burton (1979) from which the following extract is taken.

I don't want to be given pocket money, to share a room with a stranger, to have no lock on my door, to live publicly in isolation. I don't want to be bathed, dressed, wheeled, fed, entertained, all in the name of my 'happiness'. I don't want to become a client, a resident . . . but a *tenant* in a place where my physical (and perhaps mental) incapacities would be less of a nuisance to my life. A tenant in my *own* place with facilities around which made it easier for me to continue to make the decisions I (as an adult) have always made.

Yes – a place to eat sometimes – when I choose, what I choose. Yes – someone to help me with keeping my room or flat clean (like a home help). Yes – a bell to ring if I was in trouble for someone to come and help me. Yes – even a person to come and undress me and help me into bed when I ask for it (and not, if I wanted to sit up all night). And no one will decide who comes into my room but me. (And if my awful niece comes to see me I won't let *her* in!) And when I die I want to choose who sits with me or doesn't; and if I'm in no state to choose, for God's sake don't let it be my niece.

I hope I will still live with other people the way I have all my life and that they will be able to do things for me as I expect them to now. I hope there will be opportunities to change our lives the way we did at work in our union. I don't want to be isolated with twenty other residents round the edge of a big sitting room watching the children's programmes at 11 a.m. on the colour telly which matron decided *we'd* buy out of *our* amenity fund. I hope there will be people for me to give a hand to because I've spent a lot of my life doing that. And by heck, if anyone starts trying to push tenants of *our place* around we'll let them know who's running the show. (Mind you, sometimes I won't feel up to it, in which case I hope there's some other old codgers prepared to stand up for our rights.)

And no one will fetch my pension unless I say so, or have the audacity to tell me how to spend my money. *I* will pay for my meals (the ones I eat) and my contribution for my flat or room (and it had better be up to standard). The Tenants' Association at our place will need a good administrator with some assistants, some good home helps and care assistants, and we might even need to employ a community worker. Some of them will sit on our management committee.

Giving residents the right to choose increases the need for integrity on the part of staff which cannot be manufactured out of prohibitions. For example, staff may be forbidden to accept any gifts from residents, even small gifts at Christmas, technically even a glass of sherry, as I was offered by Mr Jepson. Residents need to be able to give and share.

What is essential is that both the *rights* and the *authority* of the old person are asserted. The authority of the resident refers to the recognition that the old person is an adult who has had responsibility for her life for over half a century. Staff need to support this authority and to avoid acting on an assumption that they know best whether someone should walk to keep active or needs to eat. It may well be that staff will have to support the individual's authority against that of relatives, certainly when relatives wish staff to manipulate a resident into more activity.

In this respect it is important that staff do not take all the initiatives. The old walk more slowly and they may talk more slowly. Staff may respond to this by taking over responsibility in many ways. In an earlier example I suggested that the staff initiative at admission of doing so much reinforced patterns of dependence. Staff may well assume that it is their job to start conversations, to move into a sitting room and talk to the whole group, to settle quarrels between residents. This leads only to a situation where residents are less and less able to talk to people. Staff should take *as low a profile* as possible, they are background resources, but none the less essential.

One result of this may be that residents may take a bigger part in interaction with other residents. It would seem that more privacy in the form of single rooms leads to more friendship between residents (Townsend, 1962). An increase in the residents' responsibility for their own lives may have similar beneficial outcomes.

In an earlier section I showed that some professionals would discourage the independent from entering a residential unit; alongside this Tobin and Lieberman (1976) show that the passive fare worse in the residential home. This raises two issues. First, whether the home would not benefit from a larger proportion of assertive people. There is evidence in other areas of social service provision that standards have risen partly as a result of pressure groups of consumers; in residential homes the consumers need more influence. Secondly, the home has to create situations which would allow the passive to be more masterful. There is a fine line here between forcing people to be more assertive and creating situations which *allow* that to take place. The assertive in my study used their rooms when they wished and had more possessions in them. The climate of the home must encourage others to take more initiative. Thus the home should take more assertive people and should find ways of encouraging the passive to strive for mastery.

Another factor reinforces this. The more dependent the group, the more powerful is normative control. There was abundant evidence at The Pines that expectations played a significant part in the way residents behaved. They are dependent physically but need to be encouraged to be as independent emotionally as possible so that the norms have less power.

One of the fears expressed by outsiders about living in a residential home was of loss of independence; one of the dislikes of residents was close living with people who were not their chosen friends. Consequently much of this section has been concerned with the way in which an individual may continue to control her life. In this context the word 'individual' needs emphasising. The individual should be able to live as separately as possible and therefore should be in groups as little or as much as she wishes. This will of course raise concerns for staff who may feel she should be more involved with others. 'They like to see us in the sitting rooms' said one resident, clearly because it *appears* a more purposeful way of life.

Because much present living in old age establishments takes place in groups it is sometimes assumed that the key skill is that of group work (e.g. Jones, 1979). It is not. Much of the present sitting around in groups is unwanted and unnecessary and to presume that group work is the key skill is to build on a false premise. Peace *et al.* (1979) state similarly:

The emphasis and value placed by writers on residential work upon group activities may run counter to the wishes of residents, who may not wish to be part of a group. They may prefer to be enabled to continue activities on their own or with one or two friends (a volunteer perhaps).

The central task is to enhance the *individual's* potential for mastery. Nevertheless there will be some situations where work with formal or informal groups may be appropriate. My point is that we need to escape from the picture of residential homes as group living situations.

This section has emphasised the need for residents to control their own lives. Many residents may remain unable to do this and yet still be faced by the power of the organisation. The fact that the influence is mostly exercised for good does not negate the influence. Residents may need protection from benevolent power. Each resident may need a representative who sees her point of view and will ensure her case is examined. Such a 'key person' (to use Davis's phrase, 1977) would be concerned with the interests of the individual. Lynes (1978) similarly argues the need for a sponsor for each resident.

A CONFLICT OF INTERESTS

Staff want residents to be happy. They want to provide good care for them and yet such caring may lead to dependence. Residents want to be independent and yet may enjoy some of the attention which accompanies dependence. Staff must continue to provide necessary physical care, for their task is to service the needs of the old. However, they must find a way of facing and living with the tensions that arise between caring and dependence.

Staff contact with residents is frequently at time of dependence – when residents need help to get to the lavatory, washing or bathing residents, helping them to walk. This may lead to staff judging residents by their compliance. 'She is a very pleasant old lady, *no trouble at all*' (my italics) wrote one matron about a resident who arrived at The Pines from another home. Care assistants are likely, because of the usually unskilled nature of the work, to feel undervalued; senior staff now working shorter hours may feel less involved with the whole life of the home; all staff may need escapes from continual working with people – which the office and organisational planning may supply for senior staff, and bed-making for care assistants.

In fact staff must have a clear picture of their function, and the satisfaction of their own needs must not distort the task of the establishment. For example, I have shown how staff stated that residents ought to be more active while at an unconscious level they gained satisfaction from looking after dependent people. Therefore the needs of staff – to be thanked, to be wanted, to make people happy – must be discussed in relation to the purpose of the establishment. Thus staff, aware of the range of the task and of the feelings of individuals, *must agree, as a team of workers, their approach to the running of the establishment.*

This does not mean that all residents' wishes or needs shall be met. Although residents' needs are paramount there are limits on what the organisation is able to achieve. What may be achieved depends on belief and resources. Inevitably any consideration of appropriate tasks must face the differences of interest between staff and residents. The old age home should not be a hotel with staff at hand to do everything (though many hotels in reality provide poor services and limited choice for the elderly). Hotels enhance mastery in some respects (getting others to do tasks for one) while limiting mastery in others (being less free to be oneself, having to conform to set routines). It must be a living base (or home) where staff meet the needs of residents in a way that it is agreed is appropriate.

The home should create an environment in which the needs of residents may be met. But in all this, words of caution are necessary. Most writing is by those who are not old. Most people value goals such as activity (as already shown) but alongside these the traditional virtues of self-help and independence. Mastery, as written about here, means that residents are free to choose to be dependent, and it is the job of staff to provide such services as are appropriate and viable. Two examples illustrate this.

Mr Jepson was anxious about his eneuresis. Staff might legitimately suggest various ways, including a programme to regain bladder control, which might be helpful. However, it is not their responsibility to decide that he must undergo a particular treatment.

The second example concerns fear of death. Staff should be aware of residents' possible concerns, willing to talk about them and to help resolve them. It is for residents to decide whether they wish to discuss such topics.

Chapter 13

THE OLD: ADULTS WITH RIGHTS TO SERVICES

An examination of the processes that take place in old age homes has been the major focus of this book. In the last chapter the consequences for the tasks within the institution were discussed. Now it is appropriate to return to the function that the old age home serves for the community.

In our society tensions exist for *all* the very old. They have reached an age when they must acknowledge that their dreams may not be realised; they face the increasing likelihood of sudden physical deterioration of brain or body as well as continuing and worsening chronic conditions. Less and less likely to be able to manage all aspects of their lives, they are more and more in need of services from others. Many are among the poorest and worst-housed in our society. Perhaps more of the very old feel unwanted and useless than of any other group of people. And the fact that some of the very old manage these tensions with dignity and remain loved, valued and creative does not diminish the difficulties. It needs to be remembered also that the projected numbers, absolutely and proportionately, of the very old continue to increase until the end of this century, with the result that the provision of services for this group will be one of the central social problems for the next twenty years.

It is in the context of these tensions that this book must be placed. It is in this context that despondency such as Mrs Draxton's must be viewed:

I can't sew, knit, or read; used to do all sorts of things, had prizes for needlework. The last three nights I've had to get out at night. I've seen the doctor but they just take it as a little matter. My daughter says 'What do you expect?' I look forward to breakfast. After that I sit and do nothing, that's the boring point . . . I came down from Kent to follow my daughter. I used to go to clubs, though I don't think I want to join things now. It won't be so bad when she can take me out, she used to come in and take me out.

The reasons for her sadness include her worsening physical condition, isolation from her daughter, the feeling that her concerns matter little and that life is tedious. The problems have to do with the structure of our society and are not attributable to the life-style within the old age home. The residential centre must be seen as one of the range of services available to the very old; alone it must not be expected to solve major social problems.

The old need better housing and better services. They need more houses and they need a wider variety. They need services that cross traditional boundaries, so that they may remain where possible in the type of housing of their choice with the services that they need. Thus when a residential home is faced with increasing numbers of dependent people, it should be possible to use home helps or district nurses as a temporary measure within the home. Without such a development of resources, old age homes will be used increasingly for the more dependent and there will be little opportunity for people to plan to enter a residential home at a particular age unless they go into a private or voluntary home.

Similarly the powerlessness of the old in residential units is matched by the powerlessness of the old in society at large. Both within and outside homes the old must be encouraged to assert their rights and to make demands. They need mastery of their own lives.

When that happens there will be less need for special attention to be given to those in residential centres, for the homes will reflect the wishes of the consumer. In the meantime residents and potential residents need active help in the support of their demands. Groups that assert the rights of the old in residential homes may be needed in the same way that 'Who Cares' groups have begun to do this for children.

The dilemmas of staff are paralleled by the anxieties of those who care for the old outside residential homes. For example, a woman of 85 living in her own home with considerable help from a married daughter of 60 may spend longer and longer periods of time in bed. The daughter may feel sure that staying in bed is not in her mother's best interest since the lack of exercise is leading to stiffening of the joints. How should she get the balance right between the care and direction of someone who must be allowed to decide for herself?

Thus the events within a home must be seen as a part of larger issues about ageing in our society. Yet that does not mean that the evidence accumulated in this book about processes in old age homes should be ignored. The knowledge that one of the functions carried out by such a home is to hide away some of the sadness and humiliation of the most fragile elderly, and the awareness that staff have to carry the uncertainties of other people about how best to care, must lead to clearer practice, not to disillusionment.

Indeed, one of the first steps is to reconsider the tasks of staff and the purpose of homes. By clarifying, perhaps simplifying, it becomes possible to escape from demands that can never be fulfilled and that leave everybody, residents, staff and relatives, dissatisfied. More precise statements may then be made as to what may be possible within a home.

If it is accepted that residential homes have been asked to carry some of society's uncertainties about caring for the old, then the homes are freed from some of the criticisms that are levelled against them. Yet without wide publicity, attitudes to residential homes will be slow to change. Being a resident in a home will continue to be regarded as an indication of inadequacy. Thus Mrs Williams found it hard to be a resident at The Pines since, in the past, she had visited that very home to sing to the residents. Her past picture of residents as people in need of charity made her adjustment to life in the home extremely difficult.

While the long-term task is to demonstrate the changes to those outside the homes (that facilities are vastly improved, that life within is much less restrictive), the short-term task is to make sure that this is understood by four groups of people: staff, residents, visiting professionals and neighbours. It may seem strange to head such a list with 'staff', but while many staff acknowledge improvements in care, many still consider that residential homes ought not to exist. So the purpose is to show all these groups of people that life in a residential home is not to be equated with giving up and, in particular, to ensure that prospective residents understand this.

But this statement has profound repercussions. At present demand for places in residential centres far outstrips supply but the assumption that such places should be avoided unless there is no alternative is an effective form of rationing. If living in an old age home becomes more acceptable, demand will increase dramatically.

From the broad political context I wish to return to practice within residential homes. This study illustrates some strengths and some weaknesses in practice. It has been written in the belief that homes are needed, can offer a good way of life and that weaknesses can be improved. Whatever differences there may be about the style of living that best suits old people, there are some core elements. For example, the very old are adults, with a right to choose, a right to privacy and a right to be helped. It is on these firm foundations that practice must be built and, because the very old are often weak, we need to listen carefully to what the consumers tell us about their lives. 'They'll know what it's like when they're old' mutter residents. We have to find ways of understanding the meaning of ageing and of dependence before we are old. Then staff may use that understanding to provide appropriate care. A staff member's comment from The Pines bears repetition and illustrates this well:

I sat on the floor enjoying the sun and had a chat with the men. Mr Peat is still very withdrawn but I feel he is happy in his own way. I asked him to go to the dentist but he really does not want to, he is happy chewing away with one tooth. Always get a laugh with Mr Murphy. Mr Fothergill has lost some of his spirit. I don't think he's so well.

Joe, my heart aches for him . . . I must make a point of telling the night staff he needs help in the morning . . . I really admire his courage.

APPENDIX 1: STAFF QUESTIONNAIRE

1 Job ....

2 Age 30–40...............   please tick
      41–50...............
      51–60...............
      61–70...............

3 Length of time in the home ....

4 Other similar jobs ....

5 The main reasons you took the job are (place them in order of importance with the most important at the top)
    (i) ....
    (ii) ....
    (iii) ....
    (iv) ....

6 In talking about what you do to a friend, what are the main things you
would list? (place them in order of importance with the most important
at the top)
    (i) ....
    (ii) ....
    (iii) ....
    (iv) ....

7 What qualities does a member of staff need? (place them in order of
importance with the most important at the top)
    (i) ....
    (ii) ....
    (iii) ....

8 A resident asks you to collect something from his/her room – you
have the time to do it but know he/she is fit enough to do it for him/
herself.
    Tick one answer only.
    Do you (1) Go and get it quite happily ....
            (2) Go, and think he/she is lazy ....
            (3) Say 'You are lazy today' and go ....
            (4) Say you will go and then forget ....
            (5) Say 'You can do that yourself' ....

9 What are the most rewarding parts of the job?

10 What are the most dissatisfying parts of the job?

11 Which four residents do you get on with best?
   (i) ....
   (ii) ....
   (iii) ....
   (iv) ....

12 Which four residents do you find least pleasant?
   (i) ....
   (ii) ....
   (iii) ....
   (iv) ....

13 Do you think residents should be encouraged to:
   (tick *all* those you think appropriate)
   .... Go for walks
   .... Go to the shops
   .... Go on outings
   .... Join in evening activities (e.g. film shows)
   .... Make their own beds
   .... Do some washing up
   .... Help in the kitchen (e.g. butter bread, etc.)
   .... Help other residents

14 In a few words explain why you think residents should or should not
   be encouraged to do these things.

15 If you were a resident of an old people's home what would you dislike
   the most? (place in order with the thing you dislike most at the top)
   (i) ....
   (ii) ....
   (iii) ....
   (iv) ....

16 What would be the best part of being a resident in an old people's
   home? (place in order with the thing you like most at the top)
   (i) ....
   (ii) ....
   (iii) ....
   (iv) ....

17 Look back to answers to 11 and 12. Are there any qualities or characteristics of residents that led to your choice?

18 List the most important things this home ought to accomplish.

19 What would you change if you could
   – for staff ....
   – for residents ....

20 Would you have wanted your mother to go into an old people's home?
   Yes/No
   Why?

21 Would you have wanted your father to go into an old people's home?
   Yes/No
   Why?

22 Complete the following sentences (in any way you wish):
    Residents here are . . .
    The residents ought to . . .
    Relatives of the old people are . . .
    The secret of a happy or successful old age is . . .
    Staff should not . . .

23 What type of person is best suited to life in an old people's home?

24 Would you like to live in an old people's home when you are older?
    Yes/No
    Why?

25 Which resident do you *think* you will be like when you are older?

26 Which resident would you *wish* to be like when you are older?

27 What do you most look forward to about old age?

28 What do you dread most about being old?

29 List the 10 main tasks you carry out while at the home – include any-
    thing you do with residents. Then in the columns on the right list the
    importance of the tasks as seen by (a) senior staff (b) yourself.

                                          Rank in order of importance
                                          as seen by:
                                          (a) *senior staff*   **(b)** *self*

Tasks
    1   ....
    2   ....
    3   ....
    4   ....
    5   ....
    6   ....
    7   ....
    8   ....
    9   ....
    10 ....
(Senior staff means matron and assistant matrons for care attendants,
and County Hall staff for matron and assistant matrons.)

30 What sort of behaviour would make a new member of staff un-
    popular?

31 Which 4 residents would you consider the happiest?
    (i)   ....
    (ii)   ....
    (iii) ....
    (iv)   ....

Here are some statements about old age (say 70+). Would you read each statement and put a tick in the appropriate column. If you are not sure whether you agree or disagree put a tick under '?'. Please be sure to answer every question on the list.

	Agree	Disagree	?
1 Old age is the dreariest time of life.			
2 Old age provides an opportunity to do things you've never had time for before.			
3 It's a young person's world.			
4 Families don't care about old people as they used to.			
5 Old people are best off in their own homes.			
6 It is better to keep on working till you drop.			
7 Old people have boring lives.			
8 Old people make one feel depressed.			
9 Old people should retire earlier to make way for the younger.			
10 You can be as happy when you're old as when you are younger.			
11 More money ought to be spent on keeping people out of residential homes.			
12 Old people are happiest when they have plenty to do.			
13 Old people can generally solve problems better because they have more experience.			
14 The happiest old people are those who expect to see fewer people and to do less as they age.			

Thank you for your help.

I should be grateful for any further comments you wish to make. In addition it would be helpful to have a record of some of your feelings and I have left a couple of sheets of paper for anyone who wants to do this.

Take one day – Tuesday February 22 or the nearest day you are at work to that day – and note down what you felt about particular tasks, particular attitudes of residents and staff. So you might write about things that make you angry, pleased, excited, bored, tired. And any way of writing is all right – short notes or lists of events, a diary, a poem, a few sentences – whatever you want, as long as you state which day you are writing about.

APPENDIX 2: RESIDENT INTERVIEW

---

1 Name and sex:

2 Age:
    under 60
        61–69
        71–79
        81–89
        90–99

3 Degree of mobility:
    Walks without aid
    Uses walking stick
    Uses zimmer
    Cannot walk without assistance
    Needs wheelchair

4 Mobility – performance:
    Uses public transport in town
    Walks to shops
    Walks outside home
    Does not go outside home but –
        can get to toilet on own
        can get to bed on own
        can get to meals on own

5 Drugs:
    Type:

6 Past job:
    Socio-economic class 1.
                      2.
                      3.
                      4.
                      5.

7 Spouse's past job:
    Socio-economic class 1.
                      2.
                      3.
                      4.
                      5.

8 Length of time in home (on 1 January 1977):
    under 3 months
        3–6 months
        7–12 months
        1–2 years
        2–5 years
        5+ years

9 Length of time in previous residence:
    5 years plus
    under 5 years

10 Specify places of residence in past 5 years:
    home only
    other

11 Admission process:
    Types of people involved –
        doctor
        relative
        social worker
        friend

    PROBE – how long did you think about it?
          – who suggested it?
          – to which official was first approach made?
          – which one factor made you decide to come in?

12 Relatives living:
    spouse
    brother/sister
    daughter
    son
    other of importance

13 Relatives who have died:
    spouse
    brother/sister
    daughter
    son
    other of importance

14 First impressions:
    PROBE – what did you think the home would be like?
          – what was different from what you expected?
          – how would you describe your attitude towards coming
            to the home . . .
                enthusiastic
                accepting
                resigned
                unhappy?

15 Socialisation:
   'It can't be easy getting used to a
   new home. Would you think
   about how you found out what
   to do?'

16 Purpose of old age home:
   'An old people's home ought to . . . '

17 Dependency:
   What sort of help are you most grateful for?

18 A typical day:
   Describe a typical day – PROBE.
   Look for high spots; anything that is weighted positively or nega-
   tively; any visiting other sitting areas; discussions with other residents.

19 Dependency:
   Are there some things you used to do for yourself that you need
   help with?
   List: changes since admission; types of dependency that are
   acceptable.

20 Admission and purpose:
   If you had a friend of your age would you advise them to come
   into an old people's home?

21 Aims of old age home:
   List the 3 most important things this home ought to accomplish –
   PROBE.
   Make old people happy; take over responsibilities; provide things
   for people to do; keep peace between residents.

22 Changes:
   If you were running an old people's home what sort of changes
   would you make?

23 Attitudes of staff members:
   Think about the different members of staff.
   What qualities are important?

24 Choice:
   What sorts of decisions do you make?
   What sorts of decisions can't you make that you wish you could?
   Do you like having things decided for you?
   PROBE – specify – cleaning
                     bathing
                     bed-making
                     drugs
                     meals
                     furniture
   Types of things you wish you could do?

25 Ageing:
   As people get older do they prefer to have other people to do things for them?
   Do they prefer others to make choices for them?

26 Attitudes to home:
   What do you enjoy most about being here?
   What do you like least?
   What about other residents?
   PROBE – annoying
              companionship (special friends)
              frightening
              disgusting.

27 Expectations:
   What makes a 'good' resident?
   What makes a 'bad' resident?
   PROBE – what residents think
              what staff think
   I know you are expected to tell staff if you are going to miss a meal.
   Are there other things you are expected to do?

28 Others' opinion of home:
   What do friends, relatives, outsiders tell you about coming in here, and life in the home?

BIBLIOGRAPHY

Bartak, C., and Rutter, M. (1975), 'The measurement of staff–child interaction in three units for autistic children', in Tizard, Sinclair and Clarke (1975), ch. 8.

Barton, R. (1959), *Institutional Neurosis* (Bristol: Wright).

Beedell, C. (1970), *Residential Life with Children* (London: Routledge & Kegan Paul).

Bigot, A. (1974), 'The relevance of American life satisfaction indices for research on British subjects before and after retirement', *Age and Ageing*, vol. 3.

Bowlby, J. (1951), *Maternal Care and Mental Health* (Geneva: World Health Organisation).

Brearly, C. P. (1977), *Residential Work with the Elderly* (London: Routledge & Kegan Paul).

Chown, S. (1972), 'Psychological and emotional aspects of ageing', in *Easing the Restrictions of Ageing* (Mitcham: Age Concern).

Clough, R. J. (1978a), 'Residential homes in the community', *Social Work Today*, vol. 9, no. 25.

Clough, R. J. (1978b), 'No one could call me a fussy man', *Social Work Today*, vol. 9, no. 34.

Clough, R. J. (1978c), 'Institutionalisation – not always the answer', *Social Work Today*, vol. 9, no. 43.

Clough, R. J. (1978d), 'Mastery of daily living', *Social Work Today*, vol. 10, no. 13.

Clough, R. J. (1979), 'What's in a name?', *Social Work Today*, vol. 10, no. 37.

Clough, R. J., and Burton, J. (1979), 'Rights, risks, responsibilities', *Social Work Today*, vol. 10, no. 42.

Cumming, E., and Henry, W. E. (1961), *Growing Old: The Process of Disengagement* (New York: Basic Books).

Davis, L. (1978), 'Beyond the keyworker concept', *Social Work Today*, vol. 9, no. 19.

Davies, R. M., and Duncan, B. (1975), *Allocation and Planning of Local Authority Residential Accommodation for the Elderly in Reading* (Reading: University of Reading).

DHSS (1975), *The Census of Residential Accommodation: 1970, 1. Residential Accommodation for the Elderly and the Young Physically Handicapped* (London: HMSO).

East Sussex County Council (1975), *Key Issue: The Elderly* (Lewes: East Sussex Social Services Department).

Erikson, E. (1950), *Childhood and Society* (New York: Norton).

Felstein, I. (1973), *Sex in Later Life* (Harmondsworth: Penguin).

Goffman, E. (1961), *Asylums: Essays on the Social Situations of Mental Patients and Other Inmates* (New York: Doubleday).

Goldberg, E. M. (1970), *Helping the Aged* (London: Allen & Unwin).

Goldfarb, A. (1974), 'Minor adjustments of the aged', in S. Arieti and E. Brody (eds), *American Handbook of Psychiatry, Vol. 3. Adult Clinical Psychiatry* (New York: Basic Books).

Grygier, T. (1975), 'Measurement of treatment potential', in Tizard, Sinclair and Clarke (1975), ch. 5.

Gubrium, J. F. (1973), *The Myth of the Golden Years* (Springfield, Ill.: Thomas).

Hall, P., Land, H., Parker, R., and Webb, A. (1975), *Change, Choice and Conflict in Social Policy* (London: Heinemann).

Hargreaves, D. (1972), *Interpersonal Relations and Education* (London: Routledge & Kegan Paul).

Harris, A. I. (1968), *Social Welfare for the Elderly* (London: HMSO).

Havighurst, R. J. (1963), 'Successful ageing', in R. H. Williams, C. Tibbitts and W. Donahue (eds), *Processes of Ageing*, vol. 1 (New York: Atherton Press), ch. 16, pp. 315–19.

Havighurst, R. J. (1968), 'Personality and patterns of aging', *Gerontologist*, vol. 8.

Havighurst, R. J., and Albrecht, R. (1953), *Older People* (New York: Longman).

Hendricks, J., and Hendricks, C. D. (1977), *Aging in Mass Society* (Cambridge, Mass.: Winthrop).

HMSO (1947), *Report of the Committee of Enquiry into the Conduct of Standen Farm Approved School* (London: HMSO).

HMSO (1959), *Disturbances at the Carlton Approved School*, Cmnd 937 (London: HMSO).

Hobman, D. (1977), 'The elderly', *Social Work Today*, vol. 9, no. 13.

Hughes, B., and Wilkin, D. (1980), *Residential Care of the Elderly, A Review of the Literature* (Manchester: University of Manchester).

Hunt, A. (1978), *The Elderly at Home* (London: HMSO).

Jamieson, C. (1973), 'Report for County Architect's Department' (Conrad Jamieson Associates for Cheshire Social Services).

Jeffrys, M. (1977), 'The elderly in the United Kingdom', in A. N. Exton-Smith and J. G. Evans, *Care of the Elderly: Meeting the Challenge of Dependency* (London: Academic Press), pp. 5–19.

Jones, H. (1979), *The Residential Community* (London: Routledge & Kegan Paul).

Joseph, Sir K. (1972), unpublished lecture.

Kimbell, A., and Townsend, J. (1974), *Residents in Elderly Person's Homes* (Chester: Cheshire County Council Social Services Department).

King, R. D., Raynes, N. V., and Tizard, J. (1971), *Patterns of Residential Care: Sociological Studies in Institutions for Handicapped Children* (London: Routledge & Kegan Paul).

Lambert, R. J., Millham, S. L., and Bullock, R. (1970), *A Manual to the Sociology of the School* (London: Weidenfeld & Nicolson).

Lipman, A. (1968), 'Territorial behaviour in the sitting-rooms of four residential homes for old people', *British Journal of Geriatric Practice*, June.

Lipman, A., and Slater, R. (1977), 'Homes for old people – toward a positive environment', *Gerontologist*, vol. 17, no. 2.

Lowenthal, M. J., and Boler, D. (1965), 'Voluntary versus involuntary social withdrawal', *Journal of Gerontology*, vol. 20.

Lynes, T., and Woolacott, S. (1977), 'Old people's homes – the resident as consumer', *Social Work Today*, vol. 8, no. 12.

Meacher, M. (1969), 'The future of community care', in J. Agate and M. Meacher, *The Care of the Old* (London: Fabian Society).

Meacher, M. (1972), *Taken for a Ride* (London: Longman).

Menzies, I. E. P. (1960), 'A case study in the functioning of social systems as a defence against anxiety', *Human Relations*, vol. 13.

Miller, E. F., and Gwynne, C. V. (1972), *A Life Apart* (London: Tavistock).

Millham, S. L., Bullock, R., and Cherrett, P. F. (1975a), *After Grace – Teeth* (London: Chaucer Press).

Millham, S., Bullock, R., and Cherrett, P. (1975b), 'A conceptual scheme for the comparative analysis of residential institutions', in Tizard, Sinclair and Clarke (1975), ch. 9.

Morris, P. (1969), *Put Away* (London: Routledge & Kegan Paul).

Morris, T., and Morris, P. (1963), *Pentonville* (London: Routledge & Kegan Paul).

Moss, P. (1975), 'Residential care of children', in Tizard, Sinclair and Clarke (1975), ch. 2.

National Joint Council for Local Authority Services (Manual Workers) (1980) *Handbook* (London: NJCLAS).

Neugarten, B. L., Havighurst, R. J., and Tobin, S. S. (1961), 'The measurement of life satisfaction', *Journal of Gerontology*, vol. 16.

Oxford Mail (1973), 16 October and subsequent dates.

Pain, A. (1973), 'Sharing the care at Eastwood', *Age Concern Today*, no. 7.

Peace, S. M., Hall, J. F., and Hambling, G. (1979), *The Quality of Life of the Elderly in Residential Care* (London: Polytechnic of North London).

Personal Social Services Council (1977), *Residential Care Reviewed* (London: PSSC).

Pincus, A. (1968), 'The definition and measurement of the institutional environment in homes for the aged', *The Gerontologist*, vol. 8.

Power, M. (1979), unpublished report.

Puner, M. (1974), *To the Good Long Life* (New York: Universe Books).

Righton, P. (1971), unpublished lecture.

Righton, P. (1977), 'Positive and negative aspects of residential care', *Social Work Today*, vol. 8, no. 37.

Robertson, J. (1958), *Young Children in Hospital* (London: Tavistock).

Rothman, J. (1967), *Promoting Innovation and Change in Organizations and Communities* (New York: Wiley).

Simpson, A. (1971), *The Success of Home Close: A New Design in Residential Care for the Elderly* (Cambridge: Cambridgeshire and Isle of Ely County Council Social Services Department).

Somerset County Council (1975), *Homes for the Elderly: Some Questions Answered* (Taunton: Somerset County Council Social Services Department).

Somerset County Council (1978), *Elderly Persons' Homes, Information on Residents, 1977/78* (Taunton: Somerset County Council Social Services Department).

Tizard, J., Sinclair, I., and Clarke, R. V. J. (1975), *Varieties of Residential Experience* (London: Routledge & Kegan Paul).

Tobin, S. S., and Lieberman, M. A. (1976), *Last Home for the Aged* (San Francisco: Jossey-Bass).

Townsend, P. (1962), *The Last Refuge* (London: Routledge & Kegan Paul).

Townsend, P. (1972), *The Right to Occupation* (Paris: Centre Internationale de Gerontologie Sociale).

Tunstall, J. (1966), *Old and Alone* (London: Routledge & Kegan Paul).

Whittaker, J. K. (1979), *Caring for Troubled Children* (San Francisco: Jossey-Bass).

Williams Committee (1967), *Caring for People: Staffing Residential Homes* (London: Allen & Unwin).

Wootton, B. (1959), *Social Science and Social Pathology* (London: Allen & Unwin).

INDEX

activity, assessment of 180
activity theory 5–6, 22, 169–72, 176–8, 184
admission
  allocation of places 70–2
  crisis of 196–7
  hospitalization prior to 66, 75
  people thought suited for 69–70
  planning and choice 58–9
  process of 72–5, 77–9, 168, 196–7
  reasons for 57–8, 65–9, 127–8, 188–9
  role of doctor in 64–6, 65–72
  role of social worker in 64–6, 68–9, 71–2
  types of people applying for 63
  visiting before 72–3
ageing
  attitudes to 4, 16, 31, 88, 160, 169–73, 197
  anxieties about 5, 171–2
  changing picture of self 2, 167
  influence of mobility and health 47
  in prospect 169–73
  models of 22–7
  myths of 5, 13–14
  needs and resources in 94
  patterns of 179–81
  process of 166–9
  successful 2, 5, 6–7, 13, 172, 177–8, 184, 192
anticipatory institutionalisation 18–19, 100, 157, 169
apathy 4–5, 154

Bartak 20
Barton 8
bathing 32, 89–90
Beedell 17
Bigot 34
Bowlby 8, 196
Brearley 11

care assistants 30, 40–1, 84, 141–3, 146–8
Child management scale 28
Chown 167
cleaning 84
clothing 84–5
Clough 3, 8, 14, 18, 153, 193, 196–7

community, links with 180
control 157–65
  by residents 160–1
control of life-style 22–3, 27–9, 31–3, 82–94, 163–4, 187–8
Cumming 6

daily programme 4, 32, 80–2, 85–9, 107–9, 128–9
Davies 71–2, 131
Davis 200
death 48, 117, 132, 134–8, 147, 154
departure 131–8
dependency and power 152–3, 162–3, 165, 183, 200–1
DHSS 53–6
disengagement 6, 22–3
doing things for people 153–4
domiciliary of residential care 9–13

East Sussex 55, 58, 71
emotional detachment 143, 152
Erikson 172–3, 187
Evans 56
expectations of old 167

facilities 106–7
favourites 43–4, 152
Felstein 184
furniture and decorating 33, 72–4, 93–4

Goffman 8, 19, 97–8
Goldberg 12, 14, 58, 169
gratitude 150–1
grumbling 150–1
Grygier 20
Guardian 9–10
Gubrium 5–7, 34, 94, 176, 182

Hall 31
happiness 15, 139, 141, 192
Harris 11, 57–8, 66
Haughurst 6–7, 176–7, 179–81
helping others 106, 125–6, 153–4
Hendricks 184
HMSO 107
Hobman 13
hospital 114–17, 131–3, 139
Hughes 21, 54

Hunt 51–2

incontinence 98, 111–13, 135, 159
independence 65, 112, 173, 191
indicators of life-style 28–9, 32–3
infantilising 32, 152–3, 183
institutional living
  alternative explanations 17–19
  effects of 9–10, 99–102
interviews 41–2, 118–20, 127–9, 211–14

Jamieson 9
Jeffrys 50
Jones 199
Joseph 5

Kimbell and Townsend 55–6
King 22, 28

Lambert 33, 158–9
laziness 154
life-satisfaction tests 33–4, 72, 120–1,
  128–9, 180–2
Lipman 96, 194
loneliness 70
Lowenthal 23
Lynes 200

manners 92, 99–100, 113
mapping life-style 196–7
mastery (see also control of life-style)
  195–200
Meacher 8–9, 11, 19–20, 22, 53, 190
meals 90–2, 108, 194
measurements of performance 20
medical services 32, 92–3, 125, 127
meeting physical need 194–5
Menzies 134, 136, 140
Miller and Gwynne 17, 21, 134–5, 137,
  177, 192
Millham 22, 33, 189
money 82–4
Morris, P. 8, 17
Morris, T. 8
Moss 19–20, 22
motivating residents 178

National Joint Council 146
Neugarten 34
News-sheet 41
norms 94, 159–62

old age homes
  accessibility to outside 107
  as second best 7–9

attitudes to 8–9, 118, 139–40
building programme 59
changes in practice 16
functions of 20, 190–201
goals 14–15, 139, 157, 189, 191–2
part of community 17
some national characteristics 52–60
tasks in 139–40, 143–8, 183, 193–7
title 3
typology of 22–7, 185–9
old people
  attitudes of 47–8
  demographic trends 50–3
  needs of 17, 190–1
Oxford Mail 10

pain 164
participant observation 30–1, 35, 39–41
Peace and Harding 21, 102, 149, 182,
  199–200
Personal Social Services Council 77
Pincus 21
Pines, The
  compared to all Somerset homes 60–2
  decisions about entry 72–4
  expectations in 89, 160–3, 177
  first impressions of 75–7
  indicators of life-style 82–94, 185–8
  plan 35–7
  typical day 80–2, 107–9
power 53
private boundaries 94–9, 193–4
prospectus 72, 101–2
public living 99–100
Puner 166–7, 184

questionnaires 43–4, 206–10

rejection of old 18–19, 67–8, 182
relatives 83, 118, 147, 164, 176
religion 18, 108, 111, 137, 183
reports 44–6, 77–8, 112
research 30–49
residential homes
  functions of 19–20
  models of 21–2
Residential living
  attitudes to 7–9, 17–18, 169
  changing perceptions of 38, 149–50,
  203
  gains and losses 100–4, 173–6
  pictures of good residents 100
  tasks in 104–6

residents
    adaptation to home 39–40, 182–3
    age 52–3
    dependence 53–5, 61
    interaction between sexes 162, 183–4
    marital status 55–6
    occupation 105–6
    previous residence 56–7, 61
    rooms and possessions 72–4
    services between 106, 125–6, 153–4
residents at The Pines
    Mr Arthur 162
    Mrs Barrett 159
    Mrs Black 85, 100, 155, 184
    Miss Brinton 1, 132, 162, 178
    Miss Carpenter 87, 89, 98, 100, 103,
       105, 106, 122, 123, 154, 160, 163,
       182, 186
    Miss Carrow 98
    Mrs Draxton 18–19, 30, 33, 84, 103,
       123–7, 137, 149, 162, 177, 179,
       202–3
    Miss Edwards 160–1
    Miss Ford 133
    Mr Fothergill 95, 100, 110, 113, 122,
       140, 142, 145, 159–60
    Mr Gasden 84, 90, 98, 133, 140, 142,
       149
    Miss Hackett 99, 106
    Mrs Hendon 31, 184, 187
    Mrs Hughes 84–5, 99, 123, 132, 159
    Miss Hutchins 39–40, 122, 126
    Mr Jepson 40, 98, 110–21, 123, 125,
       132–3, 137, 142, 149, 153–4, 166,
       176–7, 182–3, 198, 201
    Miss Johns 85–6, 103
    Mrs Knight 86, 87, 103, 136–7
    Mrs Loosely 97–8, 133–4, 185–6, 190
    Miss Manfield 86, 122, 126, 164–5
    Mr McNab 98, 139–40, 158
    Mr Murphy 1–2, 7, 142, 162
    Miss Napier 133–4, 158
    Mr Page 158–9
    Mr Peat 87, 99. 136, 140, 142
    Mr Peters 88. 98–9, 143
    Mrs Pinker 86, 88–9, 95, 106, 128–9,
       159, 180, 182, 186
    Mrs Quigley 89, 105–6, 163
    Mrs Richardson 65, 67. 89, 97, 99,
       102, 105–9, 124–6, 161, 182, 186

    Mrs Roberts 33–5, 89, 106, 126, 142,
       181, 185
    Mrs Sidney 85–6, 89, 90, 97, 98, 99,
       106, 160, 163
    Mrs Smith 18, 67, 87, 89, 90, 99, 106,
       122, 128–9, 133, 136–7, 142, 159,
       161, 180–1
    Mr Stevens 140, 162
    Mrs Tanner 88, 103, 142
    Mrs Tinley 133, 142, 194
    Mrs Tippitt 106, 162
    Mrs Williams 67, 90, 99, 104, 105,
       106, 121–9, 159, 160, 180–1
rewards and sanctions 158–60
Righton 11, 131
rights 197–8, 203–4
Robertson 196
Rothman 45

security 46–7, 101–2, 175, 195
segregation 162
senior staff 143–6
sexuality 184
Simpson 11
social workers see also admission
Somerset County Council 60–1, 101–2
staff, see also care assistants, senior staff
    frustrations of work 155–6
    numbers 59–60
    perspectives of 139–56
    pressures of work 139–40
    satisfactions of work 149–53, 177
    sex of 41, 148–9
stop-go regime 176–8

Tilley 15, 192
Tizard 15, 192
Tobin and Liebermann 18, 63, 67, 72,
    100, 168–9. 181, 188, 199
Townsend 8–9, 14, 22, 54–5, 57, 63–4,
    103–6, 190, 199
Tunstall 84

variables 22–3, 28

Whittaker 193
'Who Cares' 203
Williams Committee 8
Wootton 191

For Product Safety Concerns and Information please contact our EU
representative GPSR@taylorandfrancis.com Taylor & Francis Verlag GmbH,
Kaufingerstraße 24, 80331 München, Germany

Printed and bound by CPI Group (UK) Ltd, Croydon, CR0 4YY
01/05/2025
01858506-0001